Walking, it will change your life!

Chapter 1: Why Walking? Rediscovering the Power of Simple Movement

In the modern world, it's easy to forget the simplicity of walking as a form of exercise and a cornerstone of health. Yet, walking is one of the most basic human functions that connects us with our ancestors, our environment, and even our inner selves. When we walk, we engage in a natural movement that our bodies are designed to do, a movement that promotes overall well-being in ways that we often take for granted. This chapter delves into why walking remains the most effective, accessible, and underrated form of exercise in today's fast-paced, high-tech world.

The Evolution of Walking: A Natural Human Activity

Human beings have been walking for millions of years. Our early ancestors walked long distances every day to hunt, gather food, and explore new environments. In fact, walking was our primary mode of transportation for most of human history. As society advanced, we began to rely on animals and, eventually, machines to move from place to place, and walking became less of a necessity. However, our bodies never forgot. We are, in essence, designed to walk.

Walking is low-impact and gentle on the body, but it activates muscles, joints, and the cardiovascular system in ways that promote endurance, strength, and flexibility. It's the perfect exercise for all ages and fitness levels because it doesn't require any special equipment, and you can do it just about anywhere.

The Decline of Walking in Modern Life

Despite the fact that walking is one of the simplest and most effective ways to improve health, it's something many of us don't do enough of. With the advent of cars, public transportation, and sedentary jobs, our modern lifestyle has dramatically reduced the amount of walking we do daily. Instead of walking to work or to run errands, we sit for hours at desks, in cars, or on the couch. Over time, this shift has led to a rise in health problems like obesity, heart disease, and even mental health issues like depression and anxiety.

The sedentary nature of modern life has taken a toll on our overall health. Studies show that sitting for long periods can increase the risk of chronic diseases and shorten life expectancy. But just as modern life has led to less movement, the solution is surprisingly simple: walking. By adding just 4 miles of walking to your daily routine, you can counteract many of the negative effects of a sedentary lifestyle.

The Health Benefits of Walking

Walking offers a long list of benefits for both your physical and mental health. It's not just about burning calories—although that's certainly a bonus. Walking strengthens your heart, reduces the risk of cardiovascular diseases, improves circulation, and helps regulate blood pressure and cholesterol levels. It's also a weight-bearing exercise, which means it helps build and maintain strong bones, reducing the risk of osteoporosis.

Walking doesn't just benefit your body, though. It's also incredibly good for your mind. Walking can reduce stress, anxiety, and depression. It improves mood by releasing endorphins, the brain's feel-good chemicals. It also boosts brain function and helps to sharpen your memory and focus.

Here are some of the key health benefits of walking 4 miles a day:

- **Cardiovascular health**: Regular walking strengthens the heart and reduces the risk of heart disease and stroke.
- **Weight management**: Walking helps burn calories and boosts metabolism, which can aid in weight loss and maintenance.
- **Joint health**: Walking is low-impact, meaning it's gentle on the joints while still promoting flexibility and mobility.
- **Mental clarity**: Walking stimulates brain activity, improves memory, and can even reduce the risk of cognitive decline.

- **Mood enhancement**: Walking releases endorphins, which naturally improve your mood and reduce feelings of stress and anxiety.

Why 4 Miles?

You might be wondering, "Why walk 4 miles a day? Why not 3 or 5?" The answer lies in finding the perfect balance between effort, time, and results. Walking 4 miles each day strikes the right balance between being challenging enough to see significant health benefits without feeling overwhelming or unsustainable. Depending on your pace, walking 4 miles takes approximately 60 to 90 minutes. This is long enough to reap major health rewards but short enough that it can be easily integrated into even the busiest of schedules.

Four miles is also a great target for burning calories. On average, walking burns about 100 calories per mile, depending on factors such as your weight and pace. So, by walking 4 miles a day, you can burn approximately 400 calories. Over time, this can contribute significantly to weight loss or weight maintenance without the need for extreme diets or high-intensity exercise programs.

A Low-Impact, High-Reward Exercise

One of the greatest advantages of walking is that it's low-impact, meaning it doesn't put excessive strain on your joints. For those with joint pain or previous injuries, walking is a safe and effective way to stay active without risking further damage. Unlike running, which can be hard on the knees, hips, and lower back, walking provides a gentler alternative that still delivers cardiovascular and muscular benefits.

As you walk, you're not just working your legs. Walking engages your entire body, including your core and upper body. It improves your posture, balance, and coordination. And because it's low-impact, walking is an exercise you can do consistently without the need for recovery days between sessions, making it a sustainable daily practice.

The Power of Habit: Making Walking a Daily Routine

The key to unlocking the full benefits of walking lies in making it a
consistent part of your life. Walking isn't a quick fix or a temporary
solution—it's a lifelong habit that can transform your health over time.
Whether you're looking to lose weight, improve your heart health, or
simply feel more energized throughout the day, walking 4 miles a day can
help you achieve those goals.

Start by setting a realistic goal. If you're not used to walking long
distances, start with 1 or 2 miles and gradually increase your distance.
The goal is to build a routine that you can stick to, day in and day out.
The more consistent you are, the better the results you'll see. And
remember, walking is flexible—you can split your 4 miles into shorter
walks throughout the day, or you can complete it all in one session. The
most important thing is to keep moving.

Conclusion: Walking as the Foundation of Health

Walking 4 miles a day is more than just exercise—it's a lifestyle choice
that can lead to lasting health and vitality. In a world where complicated
fitness programs and high-intensity workouts are often touted as the best
way to get fit, walking stands out as a simple, effective, and sustainable
alternative. It's an exercise that's accessible to everyone, regardless of age
or fitness level.

Chapter 2: The 4 Miles Philosophy – Why It Works

The concept of walking 4 miles a day may seem simple, but it is grounded in a solid foundation of science, logic, and sustainability. Unlike extreme exercise programs that often feel unsustainable or overwhelming, the 4 Miles A Day philosophy strikes the perfect balance between effort, time, and long-term health benefits. Walking, especially for moderate distances like 4 miles, is effective, accessible, and flexible enough to fit into any lifestyle.

In this chapter, we'll explore why 4 miles is the ideal daily goal, the health advantages it provides, and how it serves as the cornerstone for a sustainable fitness routine that can last a lifetime.

Why 4 Miles? The Perfect Balance

When creating a health routine, one of the most important considerations is sustainability. Too often, people set fitness goals that are too ambitious or demanding, which leads to burnout or discouragement. High-intensity exercises may deliver results, but they often require significant effort, dedication, and recovery time. On the other hand, walking offers a more gentle, accessible way to achieve impressive health outcomes without overwhelming the body.

So why 4 miles? The number is not arbitrary. Four miles is the ideal distance because it balances several factors:

- **Time Commitment**: Walking 4 miles usually takes between 60 to 90 minutes, depending on your pace. This is manageable for most people, even those with busy schedules. You can easily split it into shorter walks throughout the day if you can't dedicate a full hour at once. Walking for this amount of time each day fits well into the average person's routine without feeling like a massive time commitment.

- **Calorie Burn**: Walking 4 miles can burn between 300 to 500 calories, depending on your weight, pace, and terrain. For most people, this is a significant number of calories to burn from a low-impact activity, and it can lead to substantial weight loss or weight maintenance over time. In fact, regular walking helps create the caloric deficit needed to lose weight without requiring extreme dieting or intense workouts.

- **Health Benefits**: Research shows that walking 30 to 60 minutes per day can lower the risk of chronic diseases, including heart disease, diabetes, and certain cancers. Walking 4 miles a day helps you meet or exceed this daily minimum recommendation for physical activity, giving you the full range of health benefits without overexerting yourself.

- **Consistency**: Unlike more intense workouts that might require recovery days, walking is something you can do every day. It's gentle on your body and joints, and it doesn't leave you feeling sore or exhausted the next day. This consistency is crucial because the key to long-term health is maintaining a regular routine over months and years—not doing something intense for a few weeks and then giving up.

The Science Behind Walking 4 Miles a Day

Walking may seem simple, but the science behind it is powerful. A consistent routine of walking 4 miles a day taps into several physiological systems in the body, providing both immediate and long-term health benefits. Here's a breakdown of what happens in your body when you walk:

- **Cardiovascular Boost**: Walking increases your heart rate and strengthens your cardiovascular system. Over time, it lowers your resting heart rate, improves circulation, and enhances your body's ability to deliver oxygen to muscles and organs. This leads to improved endurance, lower blood pressure, and a reduced risk of heart disease and stroke.

- **Metabolic Activation**: Walking 4 miles a day increases your body's metabolic rate. Your muscles require energy to move, which causes your body to burn calories during the walk and even afterward, as your metabolism stays elevated for a period of time post-exercise. The cumulative effect of daily walking promotes fat burning and weight loss, making it an excellent activity for those seeking to manage their weight.

- **Mental Health Benefits**: Walking has a profound effect on the brain. It stimulates the release of endorphins and serotonin, the "feel-good" chemicals that boost mood and reduce stress. Studies have shown that regular physical activity, such as walking, can decrease symptoms of depression and anxiety. Additionally, walking outdoors, particularly in natural environments, has been linked to enhanced creativity, better memory, and improved cognitive function.

- **Muscle and Bone Strength**: Walking is a weight-bearing exercise, meaning that your bones and muscles are supporting your body's weight as you move. This type of exercise is crucial for maintaining strong bones and muscles, particularly as we age. Walking helps prevent osteoporosis and strengthens muscles, especially in the legs, core, and hips, improving balance and stability.

- **Joint Lubrication**: One of the key reasons why walking is such a beneficial activity for people of all ages is that it helps keep your joints lubricated and flexible. As you walk, the movement promotes the circulation of synovial fluid, which lubricates the joints and reduces stiffness. This is especially important for individuals with arthritis or joint issues, as regular walking can improve mobility and decrease pain.

Consistency is Key

One of the greatest advantages of the 4 Miles A Day program is its sustainability. Walking is not an intense, high-impact exercise that requires long recovery times or special equipment. This makes it an activity you can engage in every single day, allowing for steady progress over time.

The body thrives on consistency, and small, consistent actions yield powerful results. By walking 4 miles a day, you can establish a routine that your body adapts to, promoting improved endurance, strength, and overall health.

Moreover, walking every day becomes more than just a physical activity —it can become a time for reflection, relaxation, or mindfulness. Whether you choose to walk in the morning to start your day with energy or in the evening to unwind, creating this daily ritual can become an essential part of your lifestyle.

Flexibility and Accessibility: Tailoring 4 Miles to Your Needs

Another key reason why the 4 Miles A Day philosophy works is its flexibility. Unlike many fitness programs that require a gym membership, special equipment, or specific settings, walking can be done virtually anywhere. Whether you live in a bustling city, a quiet suburb, or a rural area, walking is an activity you can incorporate into your life, no matter where you are.

- **Variety of Walking Settings**: You can walk in different environments to keep things interesting. Walk around your neighborhood, explore a local park, hike on a nearby trail, or even walk on a treadmill indoors. The flexibility of walking means you can adjust your routine to suit your preferences and needs.

- **Adjusting Pace and Intensity**: While the goal is to walk 4 miles a day, how you walk those miles is up to you. Some days, you might feel like walking at a slow, steady pace to relax and unwind. Other days, you might want to pick up the pace, turning your walk into a brisk, heart-pumping workout. You can also add intensity by incorporating hills, stairs, or intervals into your routine. The important thing is that you're moving consistently.

- **Breaking Up the Miles**: If finding a full hour to walk all at once feels challenging, don't worry! You can break up your 4 miles into smaller chunks throughout the day. For example, take a 20-minute walk in the morning, another one during your lunch break, and then finish the day with a longer walk in the evening. This flexibility makes it easier to fit walking into your schedule, regardless of how busy your day might be.

Why 4 Miles A Day is a Game-Changer

The simplicity of the 4 Miles A Day program is its greatest strength. It's a manageable distance that delivers big results, without requiring extreme effort or dedication. By committing to walk 4 miles each day, you set yourself on a path to better health, increased energy, and improved mental well-being. The cumulative benefits of walking every day extend far beyond physical fitness—they enhance your overall quality of life.

Whether you're just starting your fitness journey or looking for a way to maintain and improve your health as you age, walking 4 miles a day is a solution that can work for anyone. It's about building a routine that you can enjoy and sustain over the long term, rather than chasing short-term gains that lead to burnout.

The 4 Miles philosophy is based on consistency, accessibility, and balance. It's a program designed for longevity, and it offers a realistic, enjoyable way to make movement a part of your everyday life.

Conclusion: Walking as the Ultimate Fitness Routine

Walking 4 miles a day isn't just about reaching a number—it's about embracing a lifestyle of movement, health, and vitality. It's a philosophy that recognizes the value of consistency and the power of simplicity. Whether your goal is to improve your fitness, lose weight, or simply feel more energetic, the 4 Miles A Day approach offers a sustainable, flexible, and effective way to get there.

Chapter 3: Walking for Your Heart – Strengthening Cardiovascular Health

When it comes to heart health, walking is one of the most effective and accessible forms of exercise. Numerous studies have confirmed that regular walking significantly improves cardiovascular function, lowers the risk of heart disease, and can even reverse some of the damage caused by years of inactivity or poor lifestyle choices. Walking 4 miles a day may seem like a small commitment, but the benefits to your heart are profound and long-lasting.

In this chapter, we'll explore the science behind how walking strengthens the cardiovascular system, reduces the risk of heart-related diseases, and why walking 4 miles daily can be a key factor in maintaining and improving your heart health.

How Walking Impacts Cardiovascular Health

Your heart is a muscle, and like any muscle, it gets stronger with regular use. Walking increases your heart rate, which causes the heart to pump more blood throughout your body. This strengthens the heart over time, making it more efficient at pumping blood with each beat. As your heart becomes stronger, it can pump the same amount of blood with fewer beats, which lowers your resting heart rate. A lower resting heart rate is associated with better cardiovascular fitness and a reduced risk of heart disease.

Walking also improves circulation by dilating blood vessels, which allows for better blood flow to your muscles and organs. Improved circulation helps deliver more oxygen and nutrients to the body's tissues, enhancing overall function and promoting healing and repair.

The cardiovascular benefits of walking 4 miles a day include:

- **Increased heart strength and efficiency**
- **Improved circulation and oxygen delivery**
- **Reduced risk of heart disease and stroke**
- **Lower blood pressure**
- **Improved cholesterol levels**

Reducing the Risk of Heart Disease and Stroke

Heart disease is the leading cause of death worldwide, but regular physical activity, such as walking, can dramatically reduce your risk. Studies have shown that people who walk regularly have a 30% lower risk of heart disease compared to those who are inactive. Walking 4 miles a day helps keep your heart and blood vessels healthy by improving the elasticity of your arteries and reducing inflammation, both of which are key factors in preventing cardiovascular disease.

Walking also lowers LDL cholesterol, commonly known as "bad" cholesterol, and raises HDL cholesterol, the "good" cholesterol. High levels of LDL cholesterol contribute to the buildup of plaque in the arteries, which can lead to heart attacks and strokes. By walking regularly, you can reduce your LDL levels and prevent the accumulation of harmful plaque, thus keeping your arteries clear and your blood flowing smoothly.

Additionally, walking helps regulate blood pressure. Hypertension, or high blood pressure, is a major risk factor for heart disease and stroke. Regular walking helps lower blood pressure by making your heart more efficient and your blood vessels more flexible. The increased blood flow from walking also helps reduce the pressure on your artery walls, further lowering your risk of heart-related issues.

How Walking 4 Miles Improves Heart Efficiency

When you first start walking regularly, your heart rate increases, and you may feel out of breath as your cardiovascular system works to keep up with the demand for oxygen. Over time, however, your heart adapts to the increased activity and becomes more efficient at pumping blood. This is known as cardiovascular conditioning.

As you continue to walk 4 miles a day, your heart becomes stronger, and your body becomes more efficient at using oxygen. Your heart will not need to work as hard to pump blood, and your breathing will become more controlled. This process helps to lower your resting heart rate, meaning your heart doesn't have to work as hard when you're not exercising.

A well-conditioned heart is less prone to fatigue and stress, even during periods of physical exertion. Walking regularly also increases your lung capacity, allowing you to take in more oxygen with each breath, which further supports cardiovascular function. These improvements lead to better overall stamina and endurance, both during your walks and in everyday activities.

Walking as a Preventative Measure

One of the greatest advantages of walking for heart health is that it acts as a preventative measure against heart disease and other cardiovascular conditions. Even if you've never been diagnosed with heart disease, regular walking can reduce your risk of developing it in the future.

Walking 4 miles a day helps control other risk factors associated with heart disease, such as obesity, high blood sugar levels, and chronic inflammation. By maintaining a healthy weight through walking, you reduce the strain on your heart and lower your risk of developing conditions like diabetes, which can also negatively impact heart health.

If you've already been diagnosed with heart disease or are recovering from a heart-related event, such as a heart attack, walking is one of the

safest and most effective ways to rehabilitate your cardiovascular system.
It's a low-impact exercise that doesn't put unnecessary stress on the heart
or joints, making it an ideal choice for individuals looking to recover their
health without overexertion.

The Connection Between Walking and Blood Pressure

High blood pressure, or hypertension, is one of the most significant risk
factors for heart disease and stroke. Left unchecked, it can lead to damage
to the heart, kidneys, and brain. However, the good news is that regular
walking is an effective way to lower blood pressure naturally.

When you walk, your heart pumps more blood, which causes your blood
vessels to expand and become more flexible. This improved flexibility
reduces the pressure on the walls of your arteries, which in turn lowers
your overall blood pressure. Regular walking can help reduce both
systolic and diastolic blood pressure (the top and bottom numbers of your
blood pressure reading), bringing your levels into a healthy range.

Walking 4 miles a day can also help prevent the development of
hypertension in people who are at risk. Studies show that even moderate-
intensity exercise, like walking, can reduce the risk of developing high
blood pressure by up to 50%. And for those who already have
hypertension, walking can be a vital part of a heart-healthy lifestyle that
helps manage the condition without the need for medication or with
reduced reliance on it.

How Walking Reduces Inflammation and Promotes Heart Health

Chronic inflammation is another major contributor to heart disease. When
inflammation occurs in the blood vessels, it can damage the inner lining
of the arteries, making it easier for cholesterol to build up and form

plaques. These plaques narrow the arteries and can lead to blockages, which increase the risk of heart attacks and strokes.

Walking helps reduce inflammation by improving circulation and promoting the release of anti-inflammatory proteins. Regular physical activity also helps to regulate your body's immune response, reducing the overactive inflammatory processes that can contribute to cardiovascular disease. By walking 4 miles a day, you can reduce chronic inflammation and keep your heart and blood vessels healthy.

Maximizing the Cardiovascular Benefits of Walking

While walking is effective in its own right, there are ways to maximize its cardiovascular benefits. Here are some tips to help you get the most out of your walks:

- **Increase your pace**: Walking at a brisk pace (3.5 to 4 miles per hour) is more effective for heart health than strolling. Aim to walk fast enough that you're slightly out of breath but still able to hold a conversation. This level of intensity helps raise your heart rate and improves cardiovascular conditioning.

- **Add intervals**: Incorporate short bursts of faster walking or even light jogging into your routine. These intervals can further boost your cardiovascular health by challenging your heart to adapt to changes in intensity.

- **Walk on inclines**: Walking uphill or on varied terrain increases the intensity of your walk, which forces your heart to work harder to deliver oxygen to your muscles. This improves cardiovascular endurance and strength.

- **Use your arms**: Swinging your arms as you walk helps increase the intensity of the exercise and engages your upper body. This can raise your heart rate and improve overall circulation.

Listening to Your Heart: Monitoring Your Progress

It's important to monitor your heart health as you progress with your walking routine. One of the simplest ways to do this is by keeping track of your heart rate. Many fitness trackers and smartwatches can measure your heart rate throughout your walk, allowing you to ensure that you're walking at an intensity that benefits your heart.

You should aim to walk at about 50-70% of your maximum heart rate for moderate-intensity exercise. To find your approximate maximum heart rate, subtract your age from 220. For example, if you're 50 years old, your maximum heart rate would be around 170 beats per minute, and your target heart rate for walking should be between 85 and 120 beats per minute.

Additionally, pay attention to how you feel during and after your walks. If you experience chest pain, dizziness, or excessive shortness of breath, stop walking and consult a healthcare professional before continuing your routine.

Conclusion: Walking for a Healthier Heart

Walking 4 miles a day is one of the best things you can do for your heart. It's a simple yet powerful way to strengthen your cardiovascular system, reduce your risk of heart disease and stroke, and improve your overall health. By making walking a regular part of your life, you can enjoy the long-term benefits of a healthier heart, better circulation, and a more active, fulfilling life.

Chapter 4: Boosting Your Brain – How Walking Enhances Mental Clarity

In addition to its many physical benefits, walking 4 miles a day can have a profound impact on your mental health. Often referred to as "exercise for the mind," walking helps improve cognitive function, boost creativity, and sharpen focus. Research consistently shows that regular walking can reduce mental fatigue, enhance memory, and even protect against age-related cognitive decline.

This chapter will explore how walking benefits your brain, why it's such a powerful tool for mental clarity, and how incorporating it into your daily routine can sharpen your thinking and lift your mood.

The Mind-Body Connection: How Walking Stimulates the Brain

There is a deep, intricate connection between physical activity and mental function. When you walk, your body and brain work in harmony, engaging a complex network of muscles, neurons, and chemical processes. Physical movement triggers the release of various neurotransmitters that affect mood, concentration, and mental sharpness.

One of the key reasons walking boosts brain function is that it increases blood flow to the brain. This surge of oxygen-rich blood stimulates the production of new brain cells (a process known as neurogenesis), improves the connectivity between existing neurons, and helps repair damage caused by stress or aging. Walking also promotes the release of brain-derived neurotrophic factor (BDNF), a protein that supports the growth and survival of neurons, enhances memory, and improves cognitive function.

In addition to increasing blood flow, walking also triggers the release of endorphins and serotonin, chemicals that elevate mood and reduce feelings of stress and anxiety. This mind-body connection is one of the reasons why walking can be so effective at enhancing mental clarity, reducing brain fog, and improving overall mental well-being.

Walking and Memory: Strengthening Cognitive Function

One of the most significant benefits of walking is its positive effect on memory. Studies have shown that individuals who engage in regular physical activity, particularly walking, have better memory function and are less likely to experience age-related cognitive decline.

Walking improves memory in several ways:

- **Hippocampal Growth**: The hippocampus, a part of the brain responsible for memory and learning, often shrinks with age, leading to memory loss. However, regular walking has been shown to increase the size of the hippocampus, particularly in older adults. This growth supports better memory retention and recall.

- **Neuroplasticity**: Walking promotes neuroplasticity, the brain's ability to reorganize itself by forming new neural connections. This is crucial for learning new things, adapting to new information, and enhancing memory. The more you walk, the more you encourage your brain to adapt and grow.

- **Improved Focus and Attention**: Walking helps clear the mind and improves focus. After walking, you may notice that you're able to concentrate better, solve problems more efficiently, and recall information more easily. This boost in attention is partly due to the increased blood flow and oxygenation of the brain, which enhances cognitive function.

The Creativity Boost: Walking as a Tool for Problem Solving

Many great thinkers throughout history, from Aristotle to Steve Jobs, have been known to use walking as a way to stimulate creativity and problem-solving. And it's not just anecdotal evidence—research supports the idea that walking can enhance creative thinking.

In a study conducted at Stanford University, researchers found that walking increased creative output by an average of 60%. Participants in the study who walked, whether indoors on a treadmill or outside in nature, performed better on creative tasks compared to those who remained seated. The act of walking seems to free the mind, allowing for more divergent thinking and the generation of new ideas.

Walking allows the brain to enter a more relaxed state, which fosters creative connections and problem-solving. When you walk, especially in a non-stressful, natural environment, your mind can wander, opening up new pathways of thought that you might not access when sitting still.

Here's why walking is a powerful tool for creativity:

- **Relaxation and Divergent Thinking**: Walking puts you in a relaxed state, which is essential for divergent thinking—the process of coming up with multiple solutions or ideas. In contrast, sitting and focusing intensely on a problem can sometimes narrow your thinking. Walking breaks that cycle and allows new ideas to emerge.

- **Mind-Wandering**: The rhythmic, repetitive nature of walking encourages a state of mind-wandering, which can lead to "aha" moments and creative breakthroughs. Many people report that their best ideas come to them when they're walking, precisely because their minds are not focused on the problem at hand.

- **Environmental Stimulation**: Walking outdoors provides sensory stimulation, such as changing scenery, sounds, and smells, which can further boost creative thinking. Even walking in familiar environments can provide subtle shifts in perception that inspire new ideas.

Walking for Stress Reduction and Emotional Well-Being

Stress and anxiety are often the biggest barriers to mental clarity. When your mind is clouded with worry or tension, it's difficult to focus, think clearly, or make sound decisions. Walking offers a natural, effective way to reduce stress, clear your mind, and improve emotional well-being.

One of the reasons walking is so effective at reducing stress is that it lowers levels of cortisol, the body's primary stress hormone. Elevated cortisol levels can lead to a range of health issues, from high blood pressure to anxiety and depression. By walking regularly, you can reduce cortisol levels and promote a more balanced, calm state of mind.

In addition to lowering stress hormones, walking triggers the release of endorphins, the body's natural painkillers and mood enhancers. This "endorphin rush" helps to lift your spirits and reduce feelings of anxiety or sadness. Walking outdoors, in particular, amplifies these effects—numerous studies have shown that walking in green spaces or natural environments significantly reduces stress and improves mood compared to walking indoors or in urban settings.

Key benefits of walking for emotional well-being include:

- **Mood Enhancement**: Walking releases feel-good chemicals like serotonin and dopamine, which help improve mood and alleviate symptoms of depression.

- **Anxiety Reduction**: Walking lowers cortisol and adrenaline levels, helping to calm your mind and reduce feelings of anxiety.

- **Mindfulness and Relaxation**: Walking, especially when done mindfully, encourages relaxation and mindfulness. This can help you stay grounded, present, and focused on the positive aspects of life.

The Long-Term Cognitive Benefits of Walking

Walking isn't just a short-term solution for improving mental clarity—it has long-lasting cognitive benefits, particularly as we age. Studies have consistently shown that regular physical activity, including walking, can delay the onset of dementia and Alzheimer's disease.

As we age, our brains naturally shrink, particularly in areas responsible for memory and cognitive function. However, regular walking can slow this process and, in some cases, even reverse it. In fact, research has shown that older adults who engage in regular physical activity, such as walking, have larger brain volumes and better cognitive performance than their sedentary peers.

Walking 4 miles a day helps protect your brain in several ways:

- **Improved Blood Flow**: Walking increases blood flow to the brain, ensuring that your brain receives the oxygen and nutrients it needs to function properly and stay healthy over time.

- **Protection Against Cognitive Decline**: Walking helps preserve the hippocampus and other areas of the brain that are vulnerable to age-related decline. This can delay the onset of dementia and other cognitive disorders.

- **Neurogenesis**: Walking promotes neurogenesis, or the growth of new brain cells, which is essential for maintaining cognitive function as you age.

How to Incorporate Walking into Your Mental Health Routine

To fully experience the mental clarity and cognitive benefits of walking, it's important to approach it as part of your overall mental health routine. Here are some tips for using walking to improve your mental well-being:

- **Make walking a daily habit**: Consistency is key. Aim to walk 4 miles every day, or at least most days of the week, to experience lasting mental and emotional benefits.

- **Walk mindfully**: Instead of walking on autopilot, try to engage your senses as you walk. Notice the sounds, smells, and sights around you. Pay attention to your breathing and the rhythm of your footsteps. Walking mindfully can help reduce stress and improve focus.

- **Use walking for problem-solving**: If you're feeling stuck on a particular problem or project, take a break and go for a walk. Allow your mind to wander and see what ideas come to you as you move.

- **Walk in nature when possible**: Walking in green spaces, such as parks, forests, or by water, has been shown to have even greater mental health benefits than walking in urban environments. Try to spend time in nature to enhance your mental clarity and emotional well-being.

- **Track your mood and focus**: Keep a journal or mental note of how you feel before and after your walks. Pay attention to any improvements in mood, focus, or creativity. This can help reinforce the positive effects of walking and motivate you to keep it up.

Conclusion: Walking as a Mental Health Tool

Walking 4 miles a day is not only beneficial for your body but also for your mind. It enhances memory, boosts creativity, reduces stress, and protects against age-related cognitive decline. Whether you're looking to clear mental fog, improve your focus, or simply feel better emotionally, walking can be a powerful tool for achieving mental clarity and well-being.

Chapter 5: The Weight Loss Solution – How Walking Melts Fat

Walking is often overlooked as a tool for weight loss, but in reality, it's one of the most effective and sustainable ways to shed unwanted pounds. Unlike intense workouts that can be hard to maintain long-term, walking provides a low-impact, enjoyable form of exercise that burns calories, boosts metabolism, and supports fat loss without the need for extreme diets or strenuous training sessions.

In this chapter, we'll explore how walking 4 miles a day can help you lose weight and keep it off, why it's one of the most sustainable weight loss methods available, and how to maximize your walks for optimal fat-burning results.

How Walking Burns Calories and Fat

At its core, weight loss occurs when you burn more calories than you consume. This creates a calorie deficit, forcing your body to tap into stored fat for energy. Walking is an excellent way to achieve this calorie deficit because it burns a significant amount of calories while being gentle on your joints and muscles.

The number of calories burned during a walk depends on several factors, including your weight, pace, and terrain. On average:

- A 150-pound person burns approximately 100 calories per mile walked at a moderate pace (3 to 4 miles per hour).
- A 200-pound person burns closer to 130 calories per mile walked at the same pace.

If you walk 4 miles a day, this translates to roughly 400 to 520 calories burned, depending on your weight. Over the course of a week, that adds up to 2,800 to 3,600 calories—roughly equivalent to losing about one pound of body fat (since one pound of fat is equivalent to 3,500 calories).

Walking also increases your body's metabolic rate, meaning that you continue to burn calories even after your walk is over. This "afterburn effect," known as excess post-exercise oxygen consumption (EPOC), may not be as pronounced as it is with high-intensity workouts, but it still contributes to long-term weight loss when combined with daily walks.

Why Walking is a Sustainable Weight Loss Method

One of the biggest challenges in weight loss is maintaining progress over time. While high-intensity workouts or strict diets can help you lose weight quickly, they can be difficult to sustain in the long term, leading to burnout, plateaus, or even weight regain. This is where walking shines.

Walking is a sustainable form of exercise because it:

- **Is Low-Impact**: Unlike running or high-intensity interval training (HIIT), walking is easy on your joints and muscles. This makes it a great option for people of all fitness levels, including those with joint issues, previous injuries, or limited mobility.

- **Can Be Done Anywhere**: Whether you're walking around your neighborhood, in a park, or on a treadmill, walking is an accessible form of exercise that doesn't require a gym membership or expensive equipment.

- **Is Enjoyable**: Walking can be a social activity, a chance to enjoy nature, or a time for personal reflection. Because it's enjoyable and easy to incorporate into daily life, people are more likely to stick with a walking routine long-term.

- **Requires No Recovery Days**: High-intensity workouts often require rest days for recovery, but walking can be done every day without overloading your muscles or joints. This consistency is key to steady weight loss.

By choosing walking as your primary form of exercise, you're committing to a routine that you can maintain for the long haul. This long-term commitment is essential for sustainable weight loss and overall health improvement.

How to Maximize Fat Burning While Walking

While any walking is beneficial, there are several ways to increase the fat-burning potential of your daily walks. Here are some strategies to help you optimize your 4-mile walks for maximum weight loss:

1. **Increase Your Walking Speed**
   The faster you walk, the more calories you burn. A brisk pace (about 4 miles per hour) is ideal for fat loss because it increases your heart rate and maximizes calorie expenditure. You don't need to break into a run—just walk at a pace that makes you slightly out of breath while still allowing you to hold a conversation. This moderate-intensity level is perfect for fat burning.

2. **Incorporate Interval Training**
   Interval training involves alternating between periods of faster walking and slower walking. For example, you can walk briskly for two minutes, then slow down for one minute, and repeat throughout your walk. These intervals boost your heart rate, increase calorie burn, and help you tap into fat stores more effectively than walking at a steady pace alone.

3. **Walk on an Incline**
   Walking uphill or on an incline increases the intensity of your

walk, engaging more muscles (especially in the legs and glutes) and burning more calories. If you're walking outside, find a hilly route to incorporate inclines into your walk. If you're walking on a treadmill, adjust the incline to 5% or higher to challenge yourself.

4. **Use Weights or a Weighted Vest**
    Adding resistance to your walk, such as carrying light hand weights or wearing a weighted vest, can increase calorie burn and strengthen your muscles. However, be careful not to use weights that are too heavy, as they can strain your joints. Start with light weights and gradually increase resistance as you build strength.

5. **Track Your Steps and Distance**
    Use a fitness tracker or smartphone app to track your steps and distance during your walks. Keeping track of your progress can help you stay motivated and ensure that you're hitting your 4-mile goal each day. Aim for around 10,000 steps per day, which is roughly equivalent to 4 to 5 miles.

The Role of Walking in Targeting Belly Fat

One of the most common areas where people want to lose fat is the belly. While spot reduction (losing fat from a specific area) is a myth, walking can help reduce overall body fat, including abdominal fat, when combined with a healthy diet. Belly fat is particularly harmful because it's linked to a higher risk of cardiovascular disease, diabetes, and other health issues.

Walking helps reduce belly fat in several ways:

- **Calorie Burn**: Walking consistently creates a calorie deficit, which leads to overall fat loss. Over time, as your body loses fat, you'll notice reductions in belly fat as well.

- **Cortisol Reduction**: High levels of cortisol, the stress hormone, are linked to increased abdominal fat. Walking helps reduce stress and lower cortisol levels, making it easier to lose belly fat.

- **Improved Insulin Sensitivity**: Regular walking improves insulin sensitivity, helping your body regulate blood sugar levels more effectively. This can reduce the risk of fat storage, especially around the abdominal area.

Combining Walking with Healthy Eating for Weight Loss

While walking is a powerful tool for weight loss, it's most effective when combined with a healthy diet. The key to sustainable weight loss is creating a calorie deficit, which means burning more calories than you consume. Walking helps you burn calories, but if your diet is high in calorie-dense, low-nutrient foods, you may struggle to see results.

Here are some tips for pairing walking with a weight loss-friendly diet:

- **Focus on Whole Foods**: Build your diet around nutrient-dense, whole foods like fruits, vegetables, lean proteins, whole grains, and healthy fats. These foods provide the nutrients your body needs for energy and recovery without excess calories.

- **Watch Portion Sizes**: Even healthy foods can contribute to weight gain if eaten in large quantities. Pay attention to portion sizes and try to eat until you're satisfied, not stuffed.

- **Stay Hydrated**: Drinking plenty of water throughout the day helps support your metabolism, keep you feeling full, and maintain energy levels during your walks. Aim for at least 8 cups (2 liters) of water daily, or more if you're walking in hot weather.

- **Avoid Sugary and Processed Foods**: Processed foods, sugary snacks, and sugary drinks are often high in empty calories and can spike insulin levels, leading to fat storage. Try to limit your intake of these foods and focus on nutrient-dense options instead.

- **Eat Balanced Meals**: Make sure your meals contain a balance of protein, healthy fats, and complex carbohydrates. This will keep you feeling full and energized, preventing overeating later in the day.

Tracking Your Progress and Staying Motivated

Weight loss can be a slow and steady process, and it's important to stay motivated along the way. One of the best ways to maintain motivation is to track your progress. Keeping track of your walking routine, diet, and physical changes will help you see how far you've come and keep you focused on your goals.

Here are some ways to track your progress:

- **Keep a Walking Log**: Write down the distance, time, and intensity of each walk. You can also record how you feel during and after your walk, which can provide valuable insights into your fitness progress.

- **Measure Your Weight and Body Composition**: While weight is one indicator of progress, it's not the only one. You may find that you're losing inches around your waist or hips even if the scale isn't moving. Consider measuring your body composition (body fat percentage) or taking regular progress photos to see changes in your shape.

- **Set Milestones and Celebrate Achievements**: Break your weight loss goal into smaller, achievable milestones. Celebrate each milestone you reach—whether it's losing 5 pounds, walking a certain number of miles, or fitting into a smaller clothing size. These celebrations will help keep you motivated.

Conclusion: Walking for Weight Loss Success

Walking 4 miles a day is a powerful and sustainable way to lose weight, burn fat, and improve your overall health. By incorporating walking into your daily routine, you can create a consistent calorie deficit, boost your metabolism, and shed excess pounds without the need for extreme workouts or restrictive diets.

As you walk, remember that weight loss is a journey that requires patience and persistence. Stay consistent with your walking routine, pair it with a healthy diet, and celebrate your progress along the way. Over time, you'll not only see physical changes but also experience improved energy, mood, and well-being.

Chapter 6: Your Joints Will Thank You – Walking for Mobility

When it comes to maintaining joint health and mobility, walking is one of the best exercises you can do. Unlike high-impact activities that can put stress on your joints, walking is a low-impact, gentle form of movement that actually helps keep your joints healthy, strong, and flexible. Whether you're dealing with arthritis, recovering from an injury, or simply looking to stay active without risking joint pain, walking offers a safe and effective way to stay mobile.

In this chapter, we'll explore how walking improves joint health, supports mobility, and can even alleviate chronic joint pain. We'll also discuss practical tips for protecting your joints while walking and how to make this form of exercise accessible for individuals with joint issues.

The Anatomy of a Joint: How Walking Benefits Your Joints

Your joints are made up of several components, including cartilage, ligaments, tendons, and synovial fluid. These parts work together to allow smooth and pain-free movement. Over time, factors such as aging, injury, or inactivity can lead to joint degeneration, stiffness, and pain. The cartilage, which acts as a cushion between bones, can wear down, while ligaments and tendons may become less flexible. Walking, however, can help counteract these effects and keep your joints in good condition.

Here's how walking benefits your joints:

- **Increased Synovial Fluid Production**: Synovial fluid is a thick, slippery fluid that lubricates your joints and reduces friction between the bones. When you walk, the movement encourages the circulation of synovial fluid, which keeps your joints well-lubricated and moving smoothly. This is especially important for people with conditions like arthritis, as it helps reduce stiffness and pain.

- **Strengthened Muscles Around Joints**: Walking engages the muscles that surround and support your joints, particularly in the hips, knees, and ankles. By strengthening these muscles, walking helps to stabilize the joints and take pressure off them, reducing the risk of injury and wear-and-tear over time. Stronger muscles also improve your balance, making you less prone to falls or strains that could damage your joints.

- **Improved Range of Motion**: Walking requires a full range of motion in your legs and hips. By regularly moving your joints through their full range, you help maintain and even improve their flexibility. Over time, this increased range of motion can reduce stiffness and make daily activities easier and more comfortable.

- **Enhanced Bone Health**: Walking is a weight-bearing exercise, meaning it forces your bones to work against gravity. This helps maintain and improve bone density, which is crucial for preventing osteoporosis and other bone-related conditions that can affect joint stability. Strong bones contribute to overall joint health by providing a solid structure for muscles and tendons to work with.

Walking and Arthritis: Easing Joint Pain and Stiffness

For people with arthritis, joint pain and stiffness can make it difficult to stay active. However, walking is one of the best exercises for managing arthritis symptoms. In fact, regular walking can help alleviate pain, improve joint function, and slow the progression of the disease.

Here's why walking is beneficial for arthritis sufferers:

- **Pain Reduction**: Walking helps reduce inflammation, a major contributor to arthritis pain. It encourages the release of endorphins, the body's natural painkillers, which can reduce discomfort during and after your walk. Moreover, the movement of walking stimulates blood flow, which can reduce swelling around the joints and ease pain.

- **Improved Joint Flexibility**: Regular movement is essential for keeping joints flexible, and walking is one of the best ways to ensure that your joints stay mobile. Over time, consistent walking can reduce stiffness, making it easier to move your joints without discomfort.

- **Strengthening the Supporting Muscles**: As mentioned earlier, walking strengthens the muscles around your joints, providing better support and stability. This is particularly important for people with arthritis, as weak muscles can place additional strain on the joints, worsening symptoms.

- **Low Impact on Joints**: One of the main reasons why walking is so effective for arthritis is that it's low-impact. Unlike running or jumping, walking doesn't put excessive stress on your joints, which can exacerbate pain. This makes walking a safe and sustainable form of exercise for individuals with arthritis or joint conditions.

For individuals with severe arthritis or mobility limitations, it's important to start slowly. Walking for just 5 to 10 minutes a day can make a difference, and you can gradually build up to longer walks as your joint health improves.

The Role of Walking in Injury Recovery and Prevention

If you've ever experienced a joint injury, such as a sprained ankle or knee strain, you know how challenging recovery can be. Walking, when done correctly, can play a vital role in both injury recovery and prevention. Here's how walking can help you recover from joint injuries and prevent future ones:

- **Restoring Mobility After Injury**: After a joint injury, it's common for the joint to become stiff and lose flexibility. Walking helps gently restore range of motion and flexibility to the joint without putting too much strain on it. It's important to start with short, slow walks and gradually increase intensity and duration as the joint heals.

- **Strengthening Muscles Post-Injury**: One of the best ways to prevent future injuries is to strengthen the muscles around your joints. Walking is a simple, low-risk way to rebuild muscle strength after an injury, particularly in the legs, hips, and lower back. Strong muscles provide better support for your joints, reducing the likelihood of re-injury.

- **Improving Balance and Coordination**: Walking regularly improves your balance and coordination, which helps prevent falls and other accidents that could lead to joint injuries. This is especially important for older adults, who are at greater risk for falls and fractures.

- **Preventing Overuse Injuries**: While high-impact sports like running or basketball can increase your risk of overuse injuries (such as runner's knee or tendonitis), walking allows you to stay active without putting undue stress on your joints. By walking regularly, you can maintain joint health and prevent the wear-and-tear that often comes with more intense activities.

Tips for Protecting Your Joints While Walking

While walking is generally a low-risk activity, it's still important to take certain precautions to protect your joints and ensure that you're getting the most out of your walks without risking injury. Here are some tips for protecting your joints while walking:

1. **Wear Supportive Shoes**
   One of the most important factors in joint health while walking is wearing the right shoes. Choose walking shoes that provide adequate cushioning and support for your feet. Look for shoes with arch support, a wide toe box, and shock-absorbing soles to reduce the impact on your joints. Replace worn-out shoes regularly to ensure you're getting the support you need.

2. **Warm Up and Cool Down**
   Before you start walking, take a few minutes to warm up with gentle stretches or a slow-paced walk. This helps prepare your muscles and joints for movement and reduces the risk of injury. After your walk, cool down with a few more stretches to increase flexibility and reduce post-walk stiffness.

3. **Maintain Good Posture**
   Proper posture is key to reducing stress on your joints while walking. Keep your head up, shoulders relaxed, and your core engaged. Avoid slouching or leaning forward, as this can strain your back and hips. Walking with good posture helps distribute your weight evenly across your joints, reducing the risk of

discomfort or injury.

4. **Use Joint-Friendly Walking Surfaces**

   Whenever possible, choose softer walking surfaces, such as dirt
   trails, grass, or rubberized tracks. These surfaces are easier on
   your joints compared to hard surfaces like concrete or asphalt. If
   you're walking on harder surfaces, be mindful of your posture and
   footwear to reduce the impact on your joints.

5. **Pace Yourself**

   It's important to listen to your body and avoid overdoing it,
   especially if you have existing joint pain or are recovering from an
   injury. Start with shorter walks and gradually increase the duration
   and intensity as your joints strengthen. Don't push through pain—
   if you feel discomfort, take a break or slow down.

Walking for All Ages: Maintaining Mobility as You Age

As we age, maintaining mobility becomes increasingly important for
preserving independence and quality of life. Walking is one of the best
exercises for older adults because it promotes joint health, improves
balance, and reduces the risk of falls. Here's how walking can help people
of all ages stay mobile and active:

- **Preserving Joint Flexibility**: Regular walking helps maintain
  joint flexibility, which is essential for staying mobile as we age.
  Walking keeps your joints moving through their full range of
  motion, preventing stiffness and making it easier to perform daily
  activities like bending, reaching, and climbing stairs.

- **Preventing Falls**: Falls are a leading cause of injury in older adults, but regular walking can help prevent them. By strengthening the muscles in your legs, hips, and core, walking improves your balance and stability, making you less likely to trip or fall.

- **Improving Bone Health**: Walking is a weight-bearing exercise, which helps improve bone density and reduce the risk of osteoporosis. Strong bones are essential for maintaining mobility and reducing the risk of fractures in older adults.

For older adults or individuals with limited mobility, starting with shorter, slower walks is key. Even walking for just 10 to 15 minutes a day can make a significant difference in maintaining joint health and mobility.

Conclusion: Walking for Lifelong Joint Health

Walking 4 miles a day is one of the best things you can do for your joints. It keeps your joints lubricated, strengthens the muscles around them, and helps maintain flexibility and mobility over time. Whether you're managing arthritis, recovering from an injury, or simply looking to protect your joints as you age, walking is a safe, effective, and sustainable way to stay active and mobile.

As you continue your walking journey, remember to listen to your body and take steps to protect your joints. With the right approach, walking can become a lifelong habit that supports your overall health, well-being, and quality of life.

Chapter 7: The Stress-Buster – Walking to Improve Mental Health

In our fast-paced, constantly connected world, stress and anxiety are all too common. Many people feel overwhelmed by daily responsibilities, career pressures, and personal challenges, which can take a serious toll on mental health. While there are many strategies to manage stress, walking is one of the simplest and most effective. Not only does walking provide physical benefits, but it also has a profound impact on mental well-being, helping to reduce stress, improve mood, and foster a sense of calm.

In this chapter, we'll explore the science behind how walking reduces stress, why it's an excellent tool for managing anxiety, and how you can use walking as a regular practice to enhance your emotional well-being.

The Science of Stress Relief: How Walking Calms the Mind

When you experience stress, your body triggers a fight-or-flight response, releasing stress hormones like cortisol and adrenaline. These hormones prepare your body to deal with perceived threats, but in modern life, this response is often activated by everyday stressors such as work deadlines, financial worries, or family concerns. Over time, chronic stress can have negative effects on both your physical and mental health, contributing to anxiety, depression, high blood pressure, and even heart disease.

Walking is a powerful stress reliever because it directly counteracts the body's stress response. Here's how walking helps calm the mind:

- **Lowering Cortisol Levels**: One of the key ways walking reduces stress is by lowering cortisol, the primary stress hormone. Elevated cortisol levels are linked to anxiety, mood swings, and other stress-related issues. Walking helps reduce cortisol production, leading to a calmer, more balanced emotional state.

- **Releasing Endorphins**: Walking stimulates the release of endorphins, the body's natural "feel-good" chemicals. These neurotransmitters improve mood, reduce feelings of pain, and create a sense of well-being, often referred to as the "runner's high." Even moderate walking can trigger this endorphin release, helping you feel more positive and relaxed.

- **Boosting Serotonin Levels**: Walking also increases serotonin production, which is crucial for mood regulation. Low levels of serotonin are often associated with depression and anxiety. Regular physical activity, like walking, helps elevate serotonin levels, improving mood and reducing symptoms of anxiety and depression.

- **Regulating the Nervous System**: Walking has a calming effect on the nervous system, particularly when done in a rhythmic, mindful way. It helps activate the parasympathetic nervous system, which promotes relaxation and recovery, reducing the intensity of the body's stress response.

Walking as an Effective Tool for Anxiety Relief

Anxiety disorders are among the most common mental health conditions, affecting millions of people worldwide. While therapy and medication are effective treatments for anxiety, walking offers a natural, accessible way to manage anxiety symptoms and promote emotional balance.

Here's why walking is such an effective tool for anxiety relief:

- **Reducing Anxiety Symptoms**: Walking, especially when done outdoors in a peaceful setting, helps distract your mind from anxious thoughts and worries. The rhythmic movement of walking has a meditative quality that can help calm racing thoughts and reduce the physical symptoms of anxiety, such as rapid heart rate, muscle tension, and shallow breathing.

- **Breaking the Anxiety Cycle**: Anxiety often creates a cycle of avoidance, where people avoid activities or situations that trigger their anxiety. Walking can help break this cycle by providing a safe, controlled environment where you can confront anxious feelings in a non-threatening way. As you continue walking, you may notice that your anxiety decreases, building confidence in your ability to manage stress and anxiety.

- **Mindful Walking for Anxiety**: Walking mindfully, with a focus on your surroundings and sensations, can amplify its calming effects. By bringing attention to the present moment—how your feet feel on the ground, the sound of your breath, the sights and smells around you—you can quiet the anxious thoughts that often dominate your mind. This mindfulness helps reduce rumination, a common issue for people with anxiety.

How Walking Improves Mood and Fights Depression

Depression is a serious mental health condition that affects millions of people globally. While professional treatment is essential for managing depression, regular physical activity, including walking, has been shown to significantly improve mood and alleviate symptoms of depression.

Here's how walking supports mental health and fights depression:

- **Elevating Mood**: Walking increases levels of neurotransmitters like serotonin, dopamine, and norepinephrine, which play a key role in mood regulation. These chemicals help improve your overall emotional state, making you feel more positive and energized. Studies have shown that regular walking can be just as effective as antidepressants or psychotherapy in treating mild to moderate depression.

- **Reducing Feelings of Isolation**: Depression often leads to social withdrawal, making individuals feel isolated and disconnected. Walking provides an opportunity to get out of the house, interact with others, and connect with the world around you. Whether you walk with friends or simply greet people you pass on your route, the social aspect of walking can reduce feelings of loneliness and lift your spirits.

- **Providing a Sense of Achievement**: Depression can drain motivation and make it difficult to find joy in daily activities. Walking, however, offers a simple, manageable goal that can provide a sense of accomplishment. Completing your 4-mile walk each day, even when you're feeling down, can give you a boost of confidence and a reminder that you're taking positive steps toward improving your mental health.

Walking Outdoors: The Mental Health Benefits of Being in Nature

Walking in nature offers additional mental health benefits beyond the physical activity itself. Research shows that spending time outdoors, especially in green spaces, can reduce stress, improve mood, and enhance mental clarity. The Japanese practice of "forest bathing" (shinrin-yoku), which involves walking mindfully through a forest or natural setting, has been shown to lower cortisol levels, reduce blood pressure, and promote a sense of calm and well-being.

Here's why walking in nature is so effective at improving mental health:

- **Reducing Mental Fatigue**: Nature has a restorative effect on the mind, helping to alleviate mental fatigue caused by prolonged concentration or stress. Walking in natural environments can help refresh your mind, making you feel more alert and focused.

- **Promoting Mindfulness**: Nature walks encourage mindfulness by engaging your senses—feeling the breeze, hearing the birds, or noticing the colors of the trees and sky. This mindful engagement with the natural world helps bring you into the present moment, reducing stress and anxiety.

- **Increasing Feelings of Connection**: Walking in nature can help foster a sense of connection to something larger than yourself. Whether it's the beauty of a forest, the rhythm of the ocean waves, or the peace of a quiet park, being in nature often evokes feelings of awe and wonder, which can improve mood and provide perspective on life's challenges.

Using Walking as a Daily Stress Management Practice

Incorporating walking into your daily routine can serve as a powerful stress management tool. Whether you walk in the morning to start your day with clarity and calm or use a walk after work to decompress, walking can help you manage the stresses of everyday life in a healthy, effective way.

Here's how to make walking part of your stress management routine:

1. **Create a Daily Walking Habit**
   Consistency is key when it comes to managing stress. Try to walk at the same time each day, whether it's in the morning, during your lunch break, or in the evening. Establishing a routine will

help you build the habit of walking, making it a natural part of your day that you can rely on for stress relief.

2. **Walk with Intention**
   While any form of walking is beneficial, intentional walking for stress relief can amplify its effects. Before you start your walk, take a moment to set an intention for your walk. Maybe you want to clear your mind, release tension from your body, or focus on gratitude. Walking with intention helps align your mind and body, making the experience more therapeutic.

3. **Incorporate Breathing Exercises**
   Pairing walking with deep breathing exercises can enhance its stress-relieving effects. As you walk, try to breathe deeply and rhythmically, focusing on slow inhales and exhales. This helps calm your nervous system, reduce anxiety, and create a deeper sense of relaxation.

4. **Unplug and Disconnect**
   While it can be tempting to check your phone or catch up on emails while walking, consider leaving your devices behind or switching them to airplane mode. Disconnecting from technology allows you to fully engage with your surroundings, be present in the moment, and give your mind a break from the constant stimulation of screens.

The Long-Term Mental Health Benefits of Walking

Walking regularly offers long-term mental health benefits that go beyond immediate stress relief. Over time, walking can help build emotional resilience, improve cognitive function, and promote overall mental well-being. Here's how:

- **Emotional Resilience**: Regular physical activity like walking strengthens your ability to cope with stress. By making walking a habit, you're training your mind and body to manage stress more effectively, reducing the impact of future stressors.

- **Improved Cognitive Function**: Walking increases blood flow to the brain, which supports better cognitive function, memory, and focus. Over time, this can lead to improved mental clarity, sharper thinking, and a reduced risk of cognitive decline as you age.

- **Enhanced Self-Esteem**: Walking regularly and achieving your 4-mile goal each day can boost your self-esteem and sense of self-worth. By taking control of your mental and physical health, you'll feel more empowered and confident in your ability to manage life's challenges.

Conclusion: Walking as a Natural Stress Reliever

Walking 4 miles a day is one of the most effective and accessible ways to manage stress and improve your mental health. Whether you're dealing with anxiety, depression, or simply the stresses of daily life, walking offers a natural, healthy way to calm your mind, lift your mood, and enhance your emotional well-being.

As you incorporate walking into your daily routine, you'll likely notice improvements in both your mental and physical health. The combination of physical movement, fresh air, and mindfulness creates a powerful antidote to stress, allowing you to approach life with greater clarity, balance, and resilience.

Chapter 8: Better Sleep Starts with Walking

Sleep is essential for maintaining good physical and mental health, yet millions of people struggle with insomnia, poor sleep quality, and restlessness. Whether you have trouble falling asleep, staying asleep, or waking up feeling refreshed, walking 4 miles a day can be a game-changer for improving your sleep patterns. Numerous studies have shown that regular physical activity like walking can enhance sleep quality, help regulate circadian rhythms, and reduce the time it takes to fall asleep.

In this chapter, we'll explore the science behind how walking promotes better sleep, why it's such an effective tool for combating insomnia, and how to incorporate walking into your daily routine to optimize your rest.

How Walking Improves Sleep Quality

Sleep is a complex process that involves various biological systems, including your brain, muscles, hormones, and nervous system. Walking helps regulate these systems in ways that promote restful and restorative sleep. Here's how:

- **Regulating Circadian Rhythms**: Your body's internal clock, or circadian rhythm, plays a critical role in determining when you feel awake and when you feel sleepy. Exposure to natural light during the day helps regulate this cycle, signaling to your brain when it's time to be alert and when it's time to wind down. Walking outside, especially in the morning or early afternoon, exposes you to sunlight, which reinforces your body's natural sleep-wake cycle.

- **Reducing Sleep Onset Latency**: Sleep onset latency refers to the time it takes to fall asleep after going to bed. People who struggle with insomnia often experience prolonged sleep onset latency, spending more time awake in bed. Walking helps reduce the amount of time it takes to fall asleep by reducing stress, anxiety, and physical tension. The calming effects of walking prepare both your body and mind for rest, helping you drift off more quickly.

- **Increasing Deep Sleep**: Deep sleep, also known as slow-wave sleep, is the most restorative stage of the sleep cycle. During this phase, your body repairs tissues, strengthens the immune system, and consolidates memories. Walking can increase the amount of time you spend in deep sleep, helping you wake up feeling more refreshed and rejuvenated.

- **Improving Sleep Efficiency**: Sleep efficiency is a measure of the amount of time you spend asleep compared to the total time you spend in bed. Walking promotes better sleep efficiency by improving the quality of your sleep cycles, meaning you'll spend less time tossing and turning and more time in restorative sleep.

The Impact of Walking on Insomnia

Insomnia is one of the most common sleep disorders, affecting millions of people worldwide. Whether it's difficulty falling asleep, staying asleep, or waking up too early, insomnia can negatively impact your daily life, causing fatigue, irritability, and difficulty concentrating. While medications and therapies can be effective treatments for insomnia, walking offers a natural, non-invasive way to address the root causes of sleep problems.

Here's how walking helps combat insomnia:

- **Stress Reduction**: Stress and anxiety are major contributors to insomnia, making it difficult to relax enough to fall asleep.

Walking helps reduce stress hormones like cortisol, calming your mind and body before bedtime. A regular walking routine can also reduce overall levels of anxiety, helping you approach sleep with a more relaxed mindset.

- **Energy Expenditure**: One reason some people struggle with falling asleep is that their bodies haven't expended enough energy during the day. Walking 4 miles a day provides just the right amount of physical activity to tire your muscles and signal to your body that it's time for rest. This natural fatigue can help you fall asleep faster and stay asleep longer.

- **Balancing Hormones**: Walking promotes the production of sleep-related hormones, such as melatonin, which regulates sleep-wake cycles. Regular physical activity helps balance these hormones, making it easier to fall asleep at the right time and wake up feeling refreshed.

The Best Time to Walk for Better Sleep

While walking at any time of day is beneficial for overall health, the timing of your walk can influence its effects on sleep. Depending on your schedule and preferences, you may want to adjust the timing of your walk to maximize its impact on your sleep quality.

Here are some guidelines for when to walk for better sleep:

- **Morning Walks**: Walking in the morning is an excellent way to expose yourself to natural light, which helps regulate your circadian rhythms. Morning sunlight signals to your brain that it's time to wake up and be alert, making it easier for your body to wind down naturally at night. A brisk morning walk can also boost your energy levels and improve your mood, setting a positive tone for the rest of your day.

- **Afternoon Walks**: If you can't fit a walk into your morning routine, walking in the afternoon is another good option. Walking after lunch can help prevent the post-meal slump and keep your energy levels steady throughout the day. However, be mindful of walking too late in the afternoon—while exercise can improve sleep, vigorous activity within a few hours of bedtime can sometimes interfere with your ability to fall asleep.

- **Evening Walks**: An evening walk can be a great way to unwind after a long day and prepare your mind and body for rest. Walking in the evening helps reduce the stress and tension that may have built up throughout the day, making it easier to relax before bed. However, try to finish your walk at least two to three hours before bedtime to allow your body time to cool down and shift into sleep mode.

How Walking Helps with Sleep Disorders

In addition to insomnia, there are other sleep disorders that can disrupt your ability to get restful sleep. Walking has been shown to help manage various sleep disorders, including sleep apnea and restless legs syndrome.

- **Sleep Apnea**: Sleep apnea is a condition in which breathing repeatedly stops and starts during sleep, leading to poor sleep quality and daytime fatigue. Walking can help reduce the severity of sleep apnea by promoting weight loss and improving cardiovascular health. Excess weight, especially around the neck, is a major risk factor for sleep apnea, and regular walking can help you shed pounds and reduce airway obstruction during sleep.

- **Restless Legs Syndrome (RLS)**: Restless legs syndrome is characterized by an uncontrollable urge to move the legs, especially in the evening or during periods of rest. This can make it difficult to fall asleep or stay asleep. Walking helps reduce symptoms of RLS by improving circulation, relieving muscle tension, and providing an outlet for physical energy. Regular physical activity has been shown to alleviate the symptoms of RLS, making it easier to relax and sleep.

Walking for Better Sleep: Practical Tips

To maximize the sleep benefits of walking, it's important to incorporate walking into your routine in a way that supports your overall sleep hygiene. Here are some practical tips for using walking to improve your sleep:

1. **Consistency is Key**
   Aim to walk at the same time each day to reinforce your body's natural sleep-wake cycle. Whether it's a morning, afternoon, or evening walk, consistency helps regulate your circadian rhythm, making it easier for your body to know when it's time to sleep.

2. **Pair Walking with a Healthy Sleep Routine**
   While walking improves sleep quality, it's most effective when paired with other healthy sleep habits. Create a calming bedtime routine that includes activities like reading, meditation, or taking a warm bath. Avoid stimulants like caffeine and screens before bed to ensure that your body is fully prepared for rest.

3. **Monitor Your Walking Intensity**
    While moderate-intensity walking is great for sleep, be cautious about engaging in vigorous exercise too close to bedtime. High-intensity workouts can raise your heart rate and body temperature, making it harder to fall asleep. If you prefer to walk in the evening, opt for a leisurely stroll rather than a brisk walk.

4. **Use Walking as a De-Stressor**
    If you find yourself feeling stressed or anxious before bed, use walking as a way to release tension. A 20-minute walk in the evening can help clear your mind, calm your nerves, and prepare you for a good night's sleep. Focus on deep breathing and mindfulness during your walk to further reduce stress.

5. **Track Your Sleep Patterns**
    Consider using a fitness tracker or sleep app to monitor your sleep patterns as you incorporate walking into your routine. Tracking your sleep can provide valuable insights into how your walking routine is affecting your rest and help you make any necessary adjustments.

The Long-Term Sleep Benefits of Walking

While you may notice improvements in your sleep after just a few days of regular walking, the long-term benefits of walking on sleep quality are even more profound. Walking not only helps you fall asleep more easily but also improves the overall quality of your sleep over time. The more consistently you walk, the more likely you are to experience deeper, more restorative sleep on a nightly basis.

In addition to better sleep, walking can improve your overall health, reducing the risk of conditions that can interfere with sleep, such as obesity, sleep apnea, and high blood pressure. By making walking a regular part of your lifestyle, you'll be supporting not just your sleep but your overall well-being.

Conclusion: Walking as a Natural Sleep Aid

Walking 4 miles a day is one of the most effective natural remedies for improving sleep quality. By helping regulate your circadian rhythms, reducing stress, and promoting physical tiredness, walking sets the stage for deep, restful sleep. Whether you're struggling with insomnia or simply want to improve your sleep efficiency, walking can help you wake up feeling refreshed, energized, and ready to take on the day.

Chapter 9: Heart Health – Strengthening Your Cardiovascular System

Your heart is the engine that keeps your body running, and maintaining a healthy cardiovascular system is one of the most important things you can do to ensure long-term vitality. Fortunately, walking is one of the simplest and most effective ways to strengthen your heart. Whether you're looking to prevent heart disease, lower blood pressure, or simply improve your overall cardiovascular fitness, walking 4 miles a day can play a pivotal role in keeping your heart strong and healthy.

In this chapter, we'll explore the numerous cardiovascular benefits of walking, how it strengthens your heart and improves circulation, and why it's an excellent way to lower your risk of heart disease, stroke, and other cardiovascular conditions.

The Cardiovascular Benefits of Walking

Walking is often called a "cardio" exercise because of its ability to improve heart health and cardiovascular function. It works by increasing your heart rate, improving circulation, and helping your body more efficiently pump blood and oxygen to vital organs. Here's a closer look at the cardiovascular benefits of walking 4 miles a day:

- **Improved Heart Function**: Walking regularly strengthens your heart muscle, allowing it to pump blood more efficiently. As your heart becomes stronger, it doesn't have to work as hard to circulate blood throughout your body, which leads to a lower resting heart rate and improved heart function overall.

- **Lower Blood Pressure**: Hypertension, or high blood pressure, is a major risk factor for heart disease and stroke. Walking helps lower blood pressure by improving circulation and helping your blood vessels become more flexible, which reduces the force against your artery walls. Regular walking can significantly lower both systolic and diastolic blood pressure, making it easier to manage hypertension.

- **Increased Circulation**: Walking stimulates blood flow throughout your body, improving circulation and oxygen delivery to your muscles and organs. This improved blood flow helps keep your arteries healthy and reduces the risk of plaque buildup, which can lead to heart attacks or strokes.

- **Reduced LDL Cholesterol**: Walking can help lower levels of low-density lipoprotein (LDL) cholesterol, often referred to as "bad" cholesterol, which contributes to the formation of plaque in your arteries. At the same time, walking can raise high-density lipoprotein (HDL) cholesterol, or "good" cholesterol, which helps remove LDL from your bloodstream.

- **Better Blood Sugar Control**: Walking helps regulate blood sugar levels by improving insulin sensitivity. This reduces the risk of developing type 2 diabetes, a major risk factor for heart disease. Even short walks after meals can help your body process glucose more effectively, reducing the likelihood of blood sugar spikes.

How Walking Strengthens Your Heart

Walking is a form of aerobic exercise, meaning it increases your heart rate and breathing for an extended period of time. This sustained increase in heart rate challenges your cardiovascular system, forcing your heart and lungs to work harder to deliver oxygen-rich blood to your muscles. Over time, this regular exertion strengthens your heart muscle, improves its efficiency, and enhances its ability to pump blood throughout your body.

Here's what happens to your heart when you walk:

- **Increased Stroke Volume**: Stroke volume refers to the amount of blood your heart pumps with each beat. Regular walking increases stroke volume, meaning your heart becomes more efficient at pumping blood with fewer beats. This leads to a lower resting heart rate and better cardiovascular endurance.

- **Improved Oxygen Utilization**: Walking helps your body use oxygen more efficiently by increasing the number of capillaries (tiny blood vessels) that deliver oxygen to your muscles. As more oxygen is delivered to your muscles, your body becomes more adept at using this oxygen for energy, improving overall cardiovascular function.

- **Enhanced Heart Muscle Strength**: Just like any muscle, the heart becomes stronger with regular exercise. Walking 4 miles a day strengthens the heart muscle, making it more resilient and better able to handle periods of physical exertion or stress. A stronger heart is less likely to suffer from conditions like heart failure or arrhythmias.

- **Increased Cardiac Output**: Cardiac output refers to the amount of blood your heart pumps per minute. Walking increases cardiac output, which improves the delivery of oxygen and nutrients to your cells. This enhanced circulation helps support not only your heart but all of your body's systems, from digestion to muscle recovery.

Walking and Blood Pressure: A Natural Solution for Hypertension

High blood pressure, or hypertension, is often referred to as the "silent killer" because it rarely causes symptoms but significantly increases the risk of heart attack, stroke, and kidney disease. Fortunately, regular walking is one of the most effective lifestyle changes you can make to lower blood pressure naturally.

Here's how walking helps manage and reduce high blood pressure:

- **Improved Artery Flexibility**: Walking helps keep your blood vessels flexible and elastic, reducing the resistance to blood flow. This increased flexibility allows blood to flow more easily, lowering the pressure on your artery walls. Over time, this can lead to significant reductions in both systolic and diastolic blood pressure.

- **Reduced Resistance in Blood Vessels**: Walking helps decrease the resistance in your blood vessels, making it easier for your heart to pump blood throughout your body. This reduced resistance means that your heart doesn't have to work as hard, lowering your overall blood pressure and reducing the risk of heart-related complications.

- **Weight Management**: Excess weight is a major contributor to high blood pressure. Walking 4 miles a day can help you maintain a healthy weight, which in turn reduces the strain on your heart and blood vessels. Even moderate weight loss can lead to significant improvements in blood pressure.

- **Lower Stress Hormones**: Chronic stress is a common cause of high blood pressure. Walking helps reduce the production of stress hormones like cortisol, which can elevate blood pressure. By managing stress levels through regular walking, you can help keep your blood pressure in a healthy range.

Reducing the Risk of Heart Disease and Stroke

Heart disease and stroke are two of the leading causes of death worldwide, but regular walking can significantly reduce your risk of developing these conditions. Here's how walking 4 miles a day helps protect your heart and reduce your risk of cardiovascular disease:

- **Preventing Atherosclerosis**: Atherosclerosis is a condition in which plaque builds up in the arteries, narrowing them and restricting blood flow. Walking helps prevent atherosclerosis by improving circulation, reducing LDL cholesterol levels, and promoting the health of your blood vessels. Regular physical activity keeps your arteries clear and flexible, reducing the risk of blockages that can lead to heart attacks or strokes.

- **Maintaining Healthy Blood Vessels**: Walking stimulates the production of nitric oxide, a molecule that helps relax blood vessels and improve blood flow. This keeps your arteries healthy and reduces the risk of blood clots, which can lead to stroke.

- **Reducing Inflammation**: Chronic inflammation is a major contributor to heart disease. Walking helps reduce inflammation throughout your body by improving circulation and promoting the release of anti-inflammatory molecules. This reduction in inflammation helps protect your heart and blood vessels from damage.

- **Strengthening the Heart's Ability to Handle Stress**: Cardiovascular disease is often triggered by periods of physical or emotional stress. Walking strengthens your heart's ability to handle stress by improving its endurance and resilience. A stronger heart is better equipped to manage sudden increases in heart rate or blood pressure, reducing the risk of heart-related events.

The Role of Walking in Cholesterol Management

Cholesterol plays a significant role in cardiovascular health, and managing your cholesterol levels is crucial for preventing heart disease. Walking helps improve cholesterol levels in two key ways:

- **Lowering LDL Cholesterol**: High levels of LDL cholesterol, or "bad" cholesterol, contribute to the buildup of plaque in your arteries, increasing the risk of heart attack and stroke. Walking helps reduce LDL levels by promoting the breakdown of fat and improving your body's ability to remove excess cholesterol from the bloodstream.

- **Raising HDL Cholesterol**: HDL cholesterol, or "good" cholesterol, helps remove LDL cholesterol from your arteries and transport it to the liver for processing. Walking increases HDL levels, which improves your body's ability to clear harmful cholesterol from your bloodstream and protect your arteries from plaque buildup.

By improving your cholesterol profile, walking 4 miles a day helps maintain healthy blood vessels and reduces your risk of cardiovascular disease.

Incorporating Walking into Your Heart-Healthy Routine

To get the most cardiovascular benefits from walking, it's important to approach it as part of a heart-healthy lifestyle. Here are some tips for maximizing the heart-strengthening effects of your daily walks:

1. **Walk at a Brisk Pace**
    For maximum cardiovascular benefits, aim to walk at a brisk pace of about 3 to 4 miles per hour. This pace is fast enough to raise your heart rate and improve circulation but still manageable for most people. If you're new to walking, start at a slower pace and gradually increase your speed as your fitness improves.

2. **Add Intervals for Variety**
    To challenge your heart and improve your fitness, consider incorporating interval training into your walks. Alternate between periods of faster walking and slower walking to keep your heart rate elevated and improve cardiovascular endurance.

3. **Use Hills or Stairs**
    Walking uphill or incorporating stairs into your route increases the intensity of your walk, providing an extra challenge for your heart. The added resistance strengthens your cardiovascular system and helps burn more calories.

4. **Stay Consistent**
    The key to maintaining heart health is consistency. Aim to walk 4 miles a day, most days of the week, to keep your heart strong and reduce your risk of heart disease. Even on days when you don't feel up to a full walk, try to get some movement in to keep your heart active.

5.   **Pair Walking with a Heart-Healthy Diet**
While walking is an excellent way to strengthen your heart, it's most effective when combined with a heart-healthy diet. Focus on eating plenty of fruits, vegetables, whole grains, lean proteins, and healthy fats to support your cardiovascular system.

Conclusion: Walking for a Healthier Heart

Walking 4 miles a day is one of the best things you can do to protect your heart and improve your overall cardiovascular health. From lowering blood pressure and cholesterol to reducing the risk of heart disease and stroke, walking offers a simple, sustainable way to keep your heart strong and your arteries clear.

Chapter 10: Beating Stress – Walking as a Stress-Reduction Tool

In today's fast-paced world, stress has become a common part of daily life. Whether it's work pressures, family responsibilities, or financial concerns, chronic stress can take a serious toll on both your mental and physical health. While stress is unavoidable, finding effective ways to manage and reduce it is essential to maintaining your well-being. Walking is one of the simplest, yet most effective, tools for stress management. It not only provides physical relief but also offers significant mental and emotional benefits that help you cope with daily pressures more effectively.

In this chapter, we'll explore how walking helps reduce stress, the science behind why it works, and how to use walking as a regular practice to improve your emotional resilience and well-being.

The Physiological Effects of Stress

When you experience stress, your body triggers a physiological response known as "fight or flight." This response is designed to protect you in dangerous situations by releasing stress hormones such as adrenaline and cortisol, which prepare your body to react quickly. While this response is useful in short bursts, chronic stress can lead to harmful effects on your body, including high blood pressure, weakened immune function, anxiety, and depression.

Prolonged stress keeps your body in a heightened state of alert, which can drain your energy, disrupt your sleep, and increase the risk of developing chronic health conditions such as heart disease, diabetes, and gastrointestinal issues.

To counteract the negative effects of stress, it's important to activate the body's relaxation response, which lowers cortisol levels and promotes a sense of calm. Walking is one of the most effective ways to trigger this relaxation response and reduce the damaging effects of chronic stress.

How Walking Reduces Stress

Walking is a powerful stress-reduction tool because it addresses both the physical and mental components of stress. Here's how walking helps relieve stress:

- **Lowering Cortisol Levels**: Cortisol is the primary hormone associated with stress, and elevated cortisol levels can lead to a range of negative health effects, including weight gain, anxiety, and insomnia. Walking helps reduce cortisol levels by promoting relaxation and activating the parasympathetic nervous system, which counteracts the body's fight-or-flight response. Over time, regular walking can help lower your baseline cortisol levels, making you less reactive to stress.

- **Releasing Endorphins**: Walking stimulates the release of endorphins, the body's natural "feel-good" chemicals. These endorphins act as natural painkillers and mood enhancers, helping to reduce feelings of stress and anxiety. The endorphin rush you get from walking can create a sense of well-being and even euphoria, commonly referred to as the "runner's high."

- **Reducing Muscle Tension**: Stress often manifests as physical tension, particularly in the neck, shoulders, and back. Walking helps relieve this tension by promoting circulation and encouraging the muscles to relax. The rhythmic motion of walking can help ease tight muscles and reduce the physical symptoms of stress, such as headaches or muscle pain.

- **Boosting Mood and Energy Levels**: Chronic stress can leave you feeling fatigued and emotionally drained. Walking, however, increases circulation and oxygen delivery to your brain and muscles, which boosts energy levels and improves mental clarity. Even a short walk can help lift your mood and give you a renewed sense of focus and motivation.

Walking for Anxiety Relief

Anxiety is often tied to stress, and it can be challenging to manage when your mind is racing with worries or you feel overwhelmed by daily life. Walking offers a natural and accessible way to reduce anxiety, providing both immediate and long-term relief. Here's why walking is such an effective tool for managing anxiety:

- **Distracting Your Mind**: Anxiety often feeds on overthinking and rumination. Walking helps break the cycle of anxious thoughts by shifting your focus to your surroundings and the movement of your body. As you walk, you can immerse yourself in the sights and sounds around you, which helps quiet the noise in your mind and provides a sense of peace and distraction.

- **Promoting Mindfulness**: Walking is a great opportunity to practice mindfulness, which involves paying attention to the present moment without judgment. By focusing on the rhythm of your steps, your breathing, and your environment, you can bring your mind back to the present and away from anxious thoughts about the past or future. Mindful walking encourages a sense of calm and reduces the mental strain caused by worry.

- **Reducing Physical Symptoms of Anxiety**: Anxiety often triggers physical symptoms such as rapid heart rate, shallow breathing, and muscle tension. Walking helps mitigate these symptoms by promoting deeper breathing, increasing oxygen flow, and releasing physical tension in your muscles. As your body relaxes, your mind will likely follow suit, helping you feel calmer and more centered.

The Mental Health Benefits of Walking in Nature

While any form of walking is beneficial for stress relief, walking in nature offers even greater mental health benefits. Numerous studies have shown that spending time outdoors in natural environments can significantly reduce stress, anxiety, and depression. This practice, often called "eco-therapy" or "forest bathing," involves immersing yourself in a natural setting, such as a park, forest, or beach, to reap the healing benefits of nature.

Here's why walking in nature is so effective for stress relief:

- **Reducing Mental Fatigue**: Being in nature has a restorative effect on the mind, helping to reduce mental fatigue and improve focus. Walking in green spaces, in particular, helps shift your attention away from stressors and provides a mental break, allowing your mind to recover from the demands of daily life.

- **Lowering Cortisol Levels**: Walking in nature has been shown to lower cortisol levels more effectively than walking in urban environments. The sights, sounds, and smells of nature engage your senses and promote relaxation, which can help reduce stress hormones and induce a state of calm.

- **Increasing Feelings of Connection**: Nature has a way of making us feel connected to something larger than ourselves. Whether you're listening to the sound of birds, watching the waves crash, or admiring the beauty of a forest, walking in nature can foster a sense of awe and appreciation that reduces stress and promotes emotional well-being.

Incorporating Walking into Your Stress Management Routine

To effectively use walking as a stress-relief tool, it's important to make it a consistent part of your daily routine. Whether you walk in the morning to start your day with a sense of calm, during your lunch break to recharge, or in the evening to unwind, regular walking can help you manage stress and improve your mental health over time.

Here are some tips for incorporating walking into your stress management routine:

1. **Schedule Regular Walks**
   Consistency is key to managing stress effectively. Schedule regular walks at times that work best for your routine, such as in the morning before work, after lunch, or in the evening. Walking at the same time each day helps reinforce the habit and gives you a built-in break to de-stress.

2. **Practice Mindful Walking**
   Make your walks more effective for stress relief by practicing mindfulness as you walk. Focus on your surroundings, your breath, and the sensation of your feet hitting the ground. Engage your senses by noticing the colors, sounds, and smells around you. This mindful approach helps you stay present and reduce the mental chatter that often accompanies stress.

3. **Walk in Nature Whenever Possible**
   If you have access to a park, beach, or forest, make an effort to

walk in nature whenever you can. The calming effects of natural environments amplify the stress-relieving benefits of walking, helping you feel more grounded and connected. Even a short walk in a local park can provide a refreshing mental break.

4. **Use Walking as a Break from Technology**
   In today's digital world, we're constantly bombarded with emails, social media notifications, and online content, all of which can contribute to stress and information overload. Use your walk as an opportunity to disconnect from technology. Leave your phone behind or set it to silent mode, allowing yourself to fully engage with the present moment and take a break from the digital world.

5. **Combine Walking with Breathing Exercises**
   Deep breathing is a powerful tool for calming the nervous system and reducing stress. As you walk, try incorporating deep, rhythmic breathing exercises. Inhale slowly through your nose for a count of four, hold for a count of four, and exhale through your mouth for a count of four. This helps lower your heart rate, relax your muscles, and create a deeper sense of calm.

The Long-Term Stress Reduction Benefits of Walking

The stress-relieving benefits of walking aren't just immediate—they build over time. Regular walking not only helps you manage daily stress more effectively but also increases your emotional resilience, making it easier to handle future challenges. Over time, you'll likely notice that you feel calmer, more balanced, and better equipped to cope with life's ups and downs.

Walking also promotes overall mental health by reducing the risk of anxiety, depression, and other stress-related conditions. The endorphins released during walking create a lasting sense of well-being, while the physical activity itself provides a healthy outlet for tension and frustration. By making walking a regular part of your routine, you'll be supporting both your mental and physical health in the long term.

Conclusion: Walking for Stress Relief and Emotional Well-Being

Walking 4 miles a day is a powerful, natural way to reduce stress and improve your emotional well-being. Whether you're feeling overwhelmed by work, dealing with personal challenges, or simply seeking a way to unwind, walking offers a healthy, accessible solution for managing stress. The physical movement, combined with the calming effects of nature and mindfulness, makes walking an essential tool for anyone looking to reduce stress and enhance their quality of life.

Chapter 11: Longevity – How Walking Can Add Years to Your Life

One of the most powerful benefits of walking 4 miles a day is its potential to extend your life. Regular physical activity, especially something as simple as walking, can significantly reduce the risk of chronic diseases, improve overall health, and increase your life expectancy. As you age, maintaining an active lifestyle becomes increasingly important for staying healthy and independent. Walking is one of the most accessible ways to ensure that you stay active, healthy, and vital well into your later years.

In this chapter, we'll explore the connection between walking and longevity, how walking helps prevent chronic diseases, and why consistent walking can be one of the most effective ways to add years to your life.

The Link Between Physical Activity and Longevity

A wealth of research has shown that regular physical activity is one of the key factors in increasing lifespan. According to studies from organizations like the American Heart Association and the World Health Organization, even moderate physical activity like walking can significantly lower the risk of premature death. In fact, people who walk regularly are more likely to live longer, healthier lives compared to those who lead sedentary lifestyles.

Here's how walking promotes longevity:

- **Reducing the Risk of Chronic Diseases**: Walking helps prevent and manage a variety of chronic diseases, including heart disease, diabetes, and certain cancers. These conditions are some of the leading causes of death worldwide, and reducing your risk of developing them is crucial for extending your life.

- **Supporting Healthy Aging**: Walking helps maintain muscle mass, joint flexibility, and cardiovascular health, all of which are essential for staying active and independent as you age. Regular walking slows the natural decline in physical function that comes with aging, allowing you to maintain a higher quality of life.

- **Promoting Mental Health**: In addition to its physical benefits, walking also supports mental health by reducing the risk of depression, anxiety, and cognitive decline. A healthy mind is just as important as a healthy body when it comes to longevity, and walking helps protect both.

- **Improving Immune Function**: Walking has been shown to boost immune function, helping the body fight off infections and illnesses more effectively. A strong immune system plays a key role in longevity, particularly as you age and become more susceptible to disease.

How Walking Helps Prevent Chronic Diseases

Chronic diseases such as heart disease, diabetes, and cancer are major contributors to early death, but regular walking can significantly reduce your risk of developing these conditions. Here's a closer look at how walking helps prevent some of the most common chronic diseases:

- **Heart Disease**: Heart disease is the leading cause of death worldwide, but walking is one of the best ways to keep your heart healthy. Regular walking lowers blood pressure, reduces cholesterol levels, and improves circulation, all of which reduce the risk of heart attacks and strokes. Walking also strengthens the heart muscle, making it more efficient at pumping blood throughout the body.

- **Type 2 Diabetes**: Walking helps regulate blood sugar levels and improves insulin sensitivity, which reduces the risk of developing type 2 diabetes. For people who already have diabetes, walking can help manage the condition by stabilizing blood sugar levels and promoting healthy weight management.

- **Certain Cancers**: Research suggests that regular physical activity, including walking, can reduce the risk of developing certain types of cancer, such as breast, colon, and lung cancer. Walking helps regulate hormones, improve immune function, and reduce inflammation, all of which contribute to a lower risk of cancer.

- **Osteoporosis**: Walking is a weight-bearing exercise, meaning it forces your bones to work against gravity. This helps maintain bone density and reduces the risk of osteoporosis, a condition that weakens bones and increases the risk of fractures. Walking also improves balance and coordination, reducing the risk of falls and injuries as you age.

- **Hypertension**: High blood pressure, or hypertension, is a major risk factor for heart disease and stroke. Walking helps lower blood pressure by improving circulation and reducing the resistance in your blood vessels. Over time, regular walking can help you manage or even prevent hypertension, further protecting your heart and brain.

Improving Longevity Through Weight Management

Maintaining a healthy weight is essential for longevity, as obesity is linked to a higher risk of chronic diseases such as heart disease, diabetes, and certain cancers. Walking is one of the most sustainable ways to manage weight because it's easy to incorporate into daily life and can be done consistently over time without the need for extreme dieting or intense workouts.

Here's how walking helps with weight management:

- **Calorie Burn**: Walking burns calories and helps create a calorie deficit, which is essential for weight loss or weight maintenance. A 4-mile walk can burn between 300 and 500 calories, depending on your pace and body weight. Over time, this consistent calorie burn adds up, helping you achieve and maintain a healthy weight.

- **Boosting Metabolism**: Walking regularly boosts your metabolism, meaning your body burns more calories even at rest. This metabolic boost is particularly important as you age, when your metabolism naturally slows down. By walking regularly, you can help counteract this decline and keep your body burning calories efficiently.

- **Reducing Visceral Fat**: Walking helps reduce visceral fat, the harmful fat that accumulates around your organs and increases the risk of chronic diseases. Regular walking promotes fat loss, particularly in the abdominal area, which is crucial for preventing conditions like heart disease and diabetes.

Walking for Healthy Aging

As you age, maintaining mobility and independence becomes increasingly important for both your physical and mental health. Walking is one of the best ways to support healthy aging because it keeps your body active, strengthens your muscles and joints, and promotes mental clarity. Here's how walking helps you age gracefully and stay healthy later in life:

- **Maintaining Muscle Mass and Strength**: Walking engages the muscles in your legs, hips, and core, helping to maintain muscle mass and strength as you age. Muscle mass naturally declines with age, leading to frailty and a higher risk of falls, but regular walking can help slow this process and keep you strong and mobile.

- **Supporting Joint Health**: Walking helps keep your joints lubricated and flexible, reducing the risk of stiffness and arthritis. By moving your joints regularly, you can maintain their range of motion and prevent the aches and pains that often come with aging.

- **Improving Balance and Coordination**: Falls are a major concern for older adults, but walking helps improve your balance and coordination, reducing the risk of falls and injuries. By strengthening the muscles that support your joints and improving your proprioception (the body's ability to sense its position in space), walking helps you stay steady on your feet.

- **Boosting Cognitive Function**: Walking has been shown to improve cognitive function and reduce the risk of cognitive decline and dementia. Regular physical activity increases blood flow to the brain, which supports brain health and helps protect against conditions like Alzheimer's disease. Walking also promotes neurogenesis, the growth of new brain cells, which is essential for maintaining memory and cognitive function as you age.

Walking and Mental Health: The Key to a Longer, Happier Life

Longevity isn't just about living longer—it's also about living better. Mental health plays a crucial role in your overall quality of life, and walking can help you maintain a positive outlook and emotional well-being as you age. Here's how walking supports mental health and contributes to a longer, happier life:

- **Reducing Depression and Anxiety**: Walking helps alleviate symptoms of depression and anxiety by releasing endorphins and serotonin, the brain's natural mood boosters. Regular walking can improve your mood, reduce stress, and help you feel more connected to the world around you.

- **Enhancing Cognitive Resilience**: Walking has been shown to improve memory, focus, and mental clarity, which are important for staying sharp as you age. By promoting brain health and reducing the risk of cognitive decline, walking helps you maintain your independence and quality of life.

- **Providing a Sense of Purpose**: As people age, it's common to experience feelings of isolation or loss of purpose, especially after retirement. Walking provides a simple, structured activity that can give you a sense of accomplishment and purpose. Whether it's a daily walk around the neighborhood or a hike with friends, walking helps you stay engaged and connected.

Maximizing the Longevity Benefits of Walking

To fully experience the longevity benefits of walking, it's important to make it a regular part of your routine. Here are some tips for maximizing the impact of walking on your lifespan:

1. **Be Consistent**
   The most important factor in reaping the longevity benefits of walking is consistency. Aim to walk 4 miles a day, most days of the week, to build a regular routine that supports your heart, muscles, and mind. Even if you can't walk 4 miles every day, the key is to stay active and avoid long periods of inactivity.

2. **Vary Your Walking Routine**
   To keep walking interesting and challenging, vary your routine by walking on different terrains, such as hills, trails, or beaches. Adding variety to your walks keeps your body and mind engaged, and it can help you build strength and endurance.

3. **Combine Walking with Strength Training**
   While walking is an excellent form of cardiovascular exercise, combining it with strength training can enhance its longevity benefits. Strength training helps build and maintain muscle mass, which is essential for healthy aging. Try incorporating bodyweight exercises like squats, lunges, or push-ups into your walking routine to build full-body strength.

4. **Stay Social**
   Walking with friends, family, or a walking group adds a social element to your routine, which can improve your mental health and provide a sense of connection. Socializing during your walks also makes the activity more enjoyable, increasing the likelihood

that you'll stick with it long-term.

5. **Track Your Progress**
   Use a fitness tracker or app to monitor your steps, distance, and progress over time. Tracking your progress can help you stay motivated and see the long-term benefits of your walking routine. It also gives you a sense of accomplishment as you work toward your health and longevity goals.

Conclusion: Walking for a Long and Healthy Life

Walking 4 miles a day is one of the most effective ways to increase your life expectancy and improve your overall quality of life. By reducing the risk of chronic diseases, promoting healthy aging, and supporting mental well-being, walking offers a simple, sustainable solution for longevity. As you continue to make walking a regular part of your routine, you'll not only add years to your life but also improve the vitality and health of those years.

Chapter 12: Cholesterol and Blood Pressure – Walking for Heart Health

Maintaining healthy cholesterol and blood pressure levels is crucial for overall heart health and longevity. Elevated cholesterol and high blood pressure are two of the most significant risk factors for cardiovascular disease, leading to heart attacks, strokes, and other serious health issues. The good news is that regular physical activity—specifically walking— can help regulate both cholesterol and blood pressure, reducing the likelihood of developing these conditions.

In this chapter, we'll explore how walking 4 miles a day can help you maintain healthy cholesterol levels, lower your blood pressure, and protect your heart. You'll learn the science behind how walking benefits your cardiovascular system and practical tips to enhance these benefits.

Understanding Cholesterol and Its Role in Heart Health

Cholesterol is a waxy, fat-like substance found in your blood, and while your body needs some cholesterol to build healthy cells, having too much of it can increase the risk of heart disease. Cholesterol travels through the blood attached to proteins, forming lipoproteins. There are two types of lipoproteins that affect heart health:

- **Low-Density Lipoprotein (LDL):** Often referred to as "bad" cholesterol, LDL can build up on the walls of your arteries, forming plaque. Over time, this plaque can narrow the arteries, restricting blood flow and increasing the risk of heart attack or stroke.

- **High-Density Lipoprotein (HDL):** Known as "good" cholesterol, HDL helps remove LDL cholesterol from the arteries, transporting it to the liver for processing and removal from the body. Higher levels of HDL are protective against heart disease.

Maintaining a balance between LDL and HDL cholesterol is essential for heart health, and regular walking can help you achieve that balance.

How Walking Affects Cholesterol Levels

Walking is a proven way to improve your cholesterol profile by lowering LDL cholesterol and raising HDL cholesterol. Here's how walking influences cholesterol levels:

- **Lowering LDL Cholesterol**: Regular physical activity, such as walking, helps reduce the levels of LDL cholesterol in the blood. As you walk, your body burns fat for energy, reducing the amount of LDL cholesterol available to form plaque in the arteries. Over time, this leads to lower LDL levels and less buildup in your arteries, reducing the risk of cardiovascular disease.

- **Raising HDL Cholesterol**: Walking not only lowers bad cholesterol but also raises good cholesterol. HDL cholesterol helps remove LDL cholesterol from the bloodstream, preventing it from accumulating in the arteries. Studies have shown that moderate exercise, like walking, can raise HDL levels by as much as 10%, further protecting your heart.

- **Preventing Plaque Formation**: Walking helps improve circulation, preventing the formation of cholesterol deposits in the arteries. The increased blood flow keeps your arteries flexible and less prone to the hardening and narrowing that occurs with atherosclerosis, a condition where plaque builds up and restricts blood flow.

By walking 4 miles a day, you can make a significant impact on your cholesterol levels, reducing your risk of heart disease and promoting long-term cardiovascular health.

The Role of Blood Pressure in Heart Health

Blood pressure is the force of blood pushing against the walls of your arteries as your heart pumps blood. When blood pressure is consistently too high, it strains your heart and blood vessels, increasing the risk of heart attacks, strokes, and kidney disease. High blood pressure, or hypertension, often has no symptoms, making it a "silent killer" that can cause serious damage before it's detected.

There are two measurements that determine blood pressure:

- **Systolic Pressure**: The top number in a blood pressure reading, which measures the pressure in your arteries when your heart beats.
- **Diastolic Pressure**: The bottom number, which measures the pressure in your arteries between heartbeats, when your heart is at rest.

A normal blood pressure reading is around 120/80 mmHg. When blood pressure consistently exceeds 130/80 mmHg, it's considered elevated, and if it reaches 140/90 mmHg or higher, it's categorized as hypertension.

Walking is an effective way to keep your blood pressure within a healthy range, reducing the strain on your cardiovascular system.

How Walking Lowers Blood Pressure

Walking helps lower blood pressure in several ways, making it one of the most effective natural remedies for hypertension. Here's how it works:

- **Improving Circulation**: Walking increases blood flow throughout your body, helping to relax the blood vessels and improve circulation. This improved blood flow reduces the resistance in your arteries, making it easier for your heart to pump blood. Over time, this leads to lower blood pressure, as your heart doesn't have to work as hard to circulate blood.

- **Strengthening the Heart**: Walking strengthens the heart muscle, making it more efficient at pumping blood. A stronger heart can pump more blood with less effort, reducing the force on your arteries and lowering blood pressure. This improvement in heart efficiency is one of the key reasons why regular walkers tend to have healthier blood pressure levels.

- **Reducing Arterial Stiffness**: High blood pressure is often associated with stiffening of the arteries, which makes it harder for blood to flow freely. Walking helps keep your arteries flexible and elastic, reducing arterial stiffness and improving blood flow. This increased flexibility makes it easier for blood to flow through your arteries without causing a spike in blood pressure.

- **Promoting Weight Loss**: Excess weight is a major contributor to high blood pressure, as it puts additional strain on the heart and blood vessels. Walking helps burn calories and promote weight loss, which in turn reduces the strain on your cardiovascular system and helps lower blood pressure. Even a modest amount of weight loss can lead to significant improvements in blood pressure levels.

Walking for Better Cholesterol and Blood Pressure: Practical Tips

To fully benefit from walking's ability to improve cholesterol and blood pressure, it's important to approach your walking routine with intention. Here are some practical tips to help you optimize your walks for heart health:

1. **Walk at a Brisk Pace**
    Walking at a brisk pace of about 3 to 4 miles per hour is ideal for improving cholesterol levels and lowering blood pressure. This moderate-intensity exercise helps raise your heart rate and promote better circulation without overexertion. If you're new to walking, start with a slower pace and gradually increase your speed as your fitness improves.

2. **Incorporate Interval Training**
    To further boost the cardiovascular benefits of walking, consider incorporating interval training into your routine. This involves alternating between periods of brisk walking and slower-paced walking or even light jogging. Interval training increases your heart rate and helps improve both cholesterol levels and blood pressure more quickly than steady-state walking alone.

3. **Walk Regularly**
    Consistency is key to maintaining healthy cholesterol and blood pressure levels. Aim to walk at least 4 miles a day, most days of the week, to see lasting improvements in your heart health. Even on days when you don't feel up to a full walk, try to get in some form of movement to keep your body active.

4. **Choose Varied Terrain**
    Walking on varied terrain, such as hills or trails, adds an extra challenge to your walk, increasing its intensity and promoting

better cardiovascular health. Inclines and uneven surfaces force your heart to work harder, which can help lower blood pressure and improve cholesterol levels more effectively.

5. **Monitor Your Progress**
    Keep track of your cholesterol and blood pressure levels by scheduling regular checkups with your doctor. Many pharmacies and health centers offer free blood pressure checks, and home monitors are also widely available. Monitoring your progress can help you stay motivated and make adjustments to your walking routine as needed.

The Long-Term Benefits of Walking for Heart Health

Walking 4 miles a day offers long-term benefits for both cholesterol management and blood pressure control. Over time, consistent walking can help reduce the risk of heart disease, stroke, and other cardiovascular complications. Here's what you can expect in the long run:

- **Improved Arterial Health**: Walking helps keep your arteries clear and flexible, reducing the risk of plaque buildup and preventing atherosclerosis. Healthier arteries mean better blood flow and a reduced risk of heart attacks or strokes.

- **Lower Risk of Hypertension**: Regular walking can prevent the development of hypertension in people who are at risk. By promoting healthy circulation and improving heart efficiency, walking helps keep your blood pressure in check, even as you age.

- **Sustained Weight Loss**: Walking is one of the most sustainable forms of exercise for maintaining a healthy weight, which is crucial for long-term heart health. By preventing obesity, walking reduces the strain on your heart and helps prevent the onset of conditions like hypertension and high cholesterol.

- **Better Overall Heart Function**: A stronger, more efficient heart means less strain on your cardiovascular system, reduced risk of heart-related complications, and better overall health as you age. Regular walking helps maintain this improved heart function for years to come.

Conclusion: Walking for Lifelong Cholesterol and Blood Pressure Control

Walking 4 miles a day is one of the most effective ways to maintain healthy cholesterol and blood pressure levels, reducing your risk of heart disease and promoting overall cardiovascular health. Whether you're looking to lower your LDL cholesterol, raise your HDL cholesterol, or keep your blood pressure in a healthy range, walking offers a simple, sustainable solution.

Chapter 13: Weight Management – Walking for a Healthy Body Composition

Managing your weight is essential for overall health, longevity, and well-being. Excess body weight, particularly in the form of fat, increases the risk of a wide range of health issues, including heart disease, diabetes, joint problems, and even certain cancers. For many, weight loss can feel like an overwhelming goal, but walking 4 miles a day is one of the simplest, most sustainable, and effective ways to manage your weight long-term.

In this chapter, we'll explore how walking helps with weight management, the science behind fat burning and muscle preservation, and how you can use walking as a foundation for a healthy body composition. You'll also learn practical strategies to maximize fat loss, improve muscle tone, and maintain your results.

How Walking Promotes Weight Loss

Walking may seem like a modest form of exercise compared to intense workouts like running or strength training, but it can be just as effective—if not more so—for long-term weight management. The key is consistency and building a daily habit that is easy to maintain. Walking regularly burns calories, boosts your metabolism, and helps your body utilize fat as a fuel source.

Here's how walking contributes to weight loss:

- **Calorie Burn**: Walking burns calories by using your body's energy reserves to fuel your movements. The exact number of calories burned depends on factors like your weight, walking speed, and terrain. On average, walking 4 miles a day can burn between 300 to 500 calories. Over time, this calorie expenditure helps create a calorie deficit, which is necessary for weight loss.

- **Fat Burning**: Walking is particularly effective at burning fat. When you engage in low to moderate-intensity exercises like walking, your body uses fat as its primary energy source, especially during longer periods of activity. Regular walking helps reduce body fat, particularly around the abdomen, which is important for overall health and disease prevention.

- **Boosting Metabolism**: Walking boosts your metabolism, meaning your body burns more calories even when you're at rest. This metabolic boost continues even after your walk is over, allowing you to burn more calories throughout the day. The more regularly you walk, the more your metabolism adapts to the increased activity, making it easier to maintain or lose weight.

- **Supporting Healthy Digestion**: Walking can also aid in digestion by promoting regular bowel movements and reducing bloating. After meals, a short walk can help your body process food more efficiently, which in turn can prevent weight gain caused by poor digestion.

The Science of Fat Loss and Muscle Preservation

Effective weight management isn't just about losing weight—it's about losing fat while preserving muscle. Walking plays a vital role in achieving this balance because it encourages fat burning without breaking down muscle tissue, which often happens with more intense or restrictive exercise programs.

Here's how walking helps with fat loss and muscle preservation:

- **Low-Intensity Fat Burning**: Walking is a low-intensity exercise that predominantly uses fat as a fuel source. While high-intensity exercises like sprinting burn carbohydrates for quick energy, walking taps into your fat stores, helping you shed body fat over time. This makes walking an excellent exercise for people looking to lose fat without pushing their bodies to the extreme.

- **Muscle Preservation**: Unlike high-intensity or prolonged endurance workouts, walking is gentle on your muscles. It allows you to burn calories and fat without causing muscle breakdown, which is essential for maintaining muscle mass and strength as you lose weight. Muscle preservation is important for long-term health because muscle tissue helps support your metabolism and contributes to functional strength.

- **Toning and Strengthening Muscles**: While walking primarily burns fat, it also engages muscles in your legs, hips, and core. This regular activity helps tone and strengthen these muscle groups over time, leading to a leaner, more defined physique. Walking uphill, adding resistance with weights, or varying your terrain can further enhance muscle tone.

Walking for Sustainable Weight Management

One of the key reasons walking is so effective for long-term weight management is its sustainability. Unlike crash diets or intense workout programs that are difficult to maintain, walking is easy to incorporate into your daily life and can be done consistently for years without causing burnout.

Here's why walking is a sustainable solution for weight management:

- **Low-Impact and Joint-Friendly**: Walking is gentle on your joints and muscles, making it suitable for people of all fitness levels, including those with joint pain or injuries. Because it's low-impact, walking doesn't cause the same level of fatigue or soreness as more intense exercises, allowing you to walk daily without needing rest days.

- **Easy to Fit into Your Routine**: Walking can be done almost anywhere and at any time. Whether it's a walk around your neighborhood, a stroll during your lunch break, or a nature hike on the weekends, walking is flexible enough to fit into your schedule without disrupting your daily routine.

- **No Special Equipment Required**: Walking doesn't require a gym membership, expensive equipment, or complicated workouts. All you need is a comfortable pair of shoes and the motivation to get moving. This simplicity makes walking accessible to everyone, regardless of budget or fitness level.

- **Built-in Motivation**: Walking is an enjoyable activity that doesn't feel like a chore. Many people find walking to be a relaxing, meditative experience that helps clear the mind and reduce stress. Because it's enjoyable, you're more likely to stick with it long-term, making it an ideal form of exercise for weight maintenance.

Maximizing Fat Loss with Walking

While walking alone can promote fat loss, there are ways to maximize the fat-burning potential of your walks. By making small adjustments to your routine, you can increase your calorie burn, improve your endurance, and see results more quickly.

Here are some strategies to help you optimize your walks for fat loss:

- **Increase Your Pace**: Walking at a brisk pace increases the intensity of your workout and burns more calories. Aim to walk at a speed that makes you slightly out of breath but still allows you to hold a conversation. If you're comfortable, try power walking or incorporating short bursts of jogging to elevate your heart rate and maximize fat burning.

- **Add Intervals**: Interval training is an effective way to boost calorie burn and fat loss. Alternate between periods of brisk walking and slower walking or light jogging. For example, walk at a fast pace for 2 minutes, followed by 1 minute of slower walking, and repeat this pattern throughout your walk. Interval training challenges your cardiovascular system and helps you burn more fat in less time.

- **Incorporate Hills or Stairs**: Walking uphill or using stairs adds resistance to your walk, engaging more muscles and increasing calorie burn. If you're walking outdoors, choose routes that include hills or stairs, or use the incline feature on a treadmill to mimic the effect.

- **Carry Light Weights**: Adding resistance to your walk by carrying light hand weights or wearing a weighted vest can further increase calorie burn and help tone your muscles. However, be cautious not to use weights that are too heavy, as this can strain your joints. Start with light weights and gradually increase the resistance as your strength improves.

- **Extend Your Distance**: If you're comfortable walking 4 miles a day, consider gradually increasing your distance to challenge your body further. Adding an extra mile or two to your walk can help you burn additional calories and increase your endurance, leading to faster fat loss over time.

Walking and Diet: The Perfect Pair for Weight Management

While walking is a powerful tool for weight management, it's most effective when paired with a balanced, healthy diet. Walking helps burn calories and fat, but your diet plays an equally important role in creating a calorie deficit and providing the nutrients your body needs for energy and recovery.

Here's how to combine walking with healthy eating for optimal weight management:

- **Focus on Whole Foods**: Build your meals around nutrient-dense whole foods like fruits, vegetables, lean proteins, whole grains, and healthy fats. These foods provide the vitamins, minerals, and energy your body needs to fuel your walks and recover afterward.

- **Watch Portion Sizes**: Even healthy foods can contribute to weight gain if eaten in large quantities. Be mindful of portion sizes and aim to eat until you're satisfied, not stuffed. Controlling portions helps you maintain a calorie deficit without feeling deprived.

- **Stay Hydrated**: Drinking plenty of water is essential for both weight loss and overall health. Proper hydration supports digestion, helps regulate appetite, and prevents overeating. Aim to drink water throughout the day and carry a water bottle with you on your walks to stay hydrated.

- **Avoid Empty Calories**: Limit your intake of sugary snacks, processed foods, and high-calorie beverages, as these can quickly add up and negate the calories burned during your walk. Instead, choose nutrient-dense snacks like nuts, fruits, or yogurt to keep your energy levels steady.

Maintaining Your Results: Walking for Long-Term Success

Once you've achieved your weight loss goals, walking can help you maintain your results and prevent weight regain. Unlike extreme diets or workout programs that can be difficult to sustain, walking provides a long-term solution that fits seamlessly into your life.

Here's how to use walking for long-term weight maintenance:

- **Stay Consistent**: Consistency is key to maintaining your weight. Continue walking 4 miles a day, even after you've reached your weight loss goals, to keep your metabolism active and prevent weight gain. Walking regularly will help you stay lean, fit, and healthy over the long term.

- **Monitor Your Progress**: Keep track of your weight, body measurements, and fitness levels to stay on top of your progress. Regular monitoring helps you catch any fluctuations early and make adjustments to your walking routine or diet as needed.

- **Adjust as Needed**: If you notice that your weight is creeping up, increase the intensity or duration of your walks to burn more calories. Walking more frequently, adding distance, or incorporating intervals can help you get back on track and maintain your desired weight.

Conclusion: Walking for a Healthy Body Composition

Walking 4 miles a day is a simple, sustainable, and highly effective way to manage your weight, burn fat, and improve your overall body composition. Whether your goal is to lose weight, tone your muscles, or maintain a healthy weight long-term, walking provides the perfect foundation for a balanced approach to fitness.

Chapter 14: Walking for Better Sleep – How Physical Activity Improves Rest

In our modern, fast-paced world, getting a good night's sleep can often seem elusive. Insomnia, restless nights, and poor sleep quality can affect our physical and mental health, leaving us feeling fatigued, unfocused, and stressed. Walking 4 miles a day, however, offers a natural and effective solution for improving sleep. Regular physical activity like walking not only helps you fall asleep faster but also enhances the quality of your sleep, allowing you to wake up feeling refreshed and rejuvenated.

In this chapter, we'll explore the science behind how walking improves sleep, why it's so effective for combating insomnia and sleep disturbances, and how you can incorporate walking into your routine to optimize your rest.

The Importance of Sleep for Health and Well-Being

Sleep is essential for overall health and well-being. It's during sleep that our bodies and minds rest, recover, and repair, ensuring we are prepared for the next day. Poor sleep, on the other hand, can have far-reaching effects on our health, including:

- **Increased Stress**: Lack of sleep raises cortisol levels, which leads to higher stress levels. Over time, this can cause chronic stress, anxiety, and irritability.

- **Weakened Immune System**: Sleep is critical for maintaining a healthy immune system. People who don't get enough sleep are more susceptible to illness and have a harder time fighting off infections.

- **Weight Gain**: Poor sleep disrupts hormones that regulate hunger and appetite, leading to overeating and weight gain. This hormonal imbalance also makes it harder for the body to process fat and glucose effectively.

- **Cognitive Decline**: Sleep is essential for memory consolidation and cognitive function. Without adequate rest, it's harder to concentrate, think clearly, and retain new information.

The good news is that regular walking can directly impact sleep quality, helping you get the restorative rest your body and mind need.

How Walking Improves Sleep Quality

Walking positively impacts sleep in several ways, making it one of the most effective forms of physical activity for improving both the duration and quality of sleep. Here's how walking helps promote better sleep:

- **Regulating Circadian Rhythms**: Your body's circadian rhythm is the internal clock that regulates your sleep-wake cycle. Exposure to natural light during the day is a key factor in maintaining this rhythm, signaling to your brain when it's time to be awake and when it's time to sleep. Walking outdoors during daylight hours, particularly in the morning or early afternoon, helps reset your circadian rhythm, making it easier to fall asleep and wake up at consistent times.

- **Reducing Sleep Onset Latency**: Sleep onset latency refers to how long it takes you to fall asleep after going to bed. Many people with insomnia or sleep disturbances spend long periods lying awake, trying to drift off. Walking helps reduce sleep onset latency by promoting relaxation and reducing anxiety. As a low-impact exercise, walking helps your body release built-up energy and tension, making it easier to fall asleep quickly when you go to bed.

- **Promoting Deep Sleep**: Deep sleep, also known as slow-wave sleep, is the most restorative phase of the sleep cycle. During deep sleep, your body repairs tissues, builds bone and muscle, and strengthens the immune system. Walking increases the time spent in deep sleep, improving the quality of your rest and helping you wake up feeling more refreshed.

- **Improving Sleep Efficiency**: Sleep efficiency refers to the amount of time you spend asleep compared to the time you spend in bed. People who struggle with sleep often experience low sleep efficiency, meaning they spend a lot of time in bed without actually sleeping. Walking helps improve sleep efficiency by ensuring that the time you spend in bed is more restful, with fewer interruptions or awakenings.

Walking as a Natural Remedy for Insomnia

Insomnia is one of the most common sleep disorders, affecting millions of people around the world. Whether it's difficulty falling asleep, staying asleep, or waking up too early, insomnia can significantly affect your quality of life. While medications and therapies can help, walking offers a natural, non-invasive way to address the root causes of insomnia and improve sleep.

Here's how walking helps alleviate insomnia:

- **Reducing Stress and Anxiety**: Stress and anxiety are major contributors to insomnia. Walking helps lower cortisol levels and promotes the release of endorphins, which are natural mood boosters. This reduction in stress and anxiety makes it easier for your mind and body to relax before bedtime, increasing your chances of falling asleep quickly and staying asleep throughout the night.

- **Physical Fatigue**: Insomnia can sometimes result from a lack of physical activity during the day. Walking helps tire your body naturally, creating physical fatigue that encourages deeper, more restful sleep. By walking regularly, you engage your muscles and expend energy, making it easier for your body to relax and recover when it's time to sleep.

- **Balancing Hormones**: Walking helps regulate the production of hormones that affect sleep, such as melatonin. Melatonin is the hormone that controls your sleep-wake cycle, and walking during daylight hours helps boost its production at night, improving your ability to fall asleep and stay asleep.

The Best Time to Walk for Better Sleep

While walking at any time of day can improve sleep quality, the timing of your walks can influence their effect on your sleep patterns. Depending on your schedule and preferences, you can adjust the timing of your walks to suit your sleep needs.

Here are some guidelines for when to walk to maximize the sleep benefits:

- **Morning Walks**: Walking in the morning is ideal for regulating your circadian rhythm and helping you wake up feeling energized. Morning sunlight reinforces your body's natural sleep-wake cycle, signaling to your brain that it's time to be alert and awake. This can help you feel more tired in the evening when it's time to wind down, leading to better sleep at night.

- **Afternoon Walks**: If you're unable to walk in the morning, an afternoon walk can also help improve sleep. Walking after lunch can prevent the post-meal slump and keep your energy levels stable throughout the day. Just be mindful not to walk too close to bedtime, as late-afternoon or evening exercise can sometimes be too stimulating, making it harder to fall asleep.

- **Evening Walks**: A gentle evening walk can be a great way to relax and unwind after a busy day. Walking in the evening helps release tension from your body, allowing you to transition smoothly into a restful sleep. However, try to finish your walk at least two to three hours before bed to give your body time to cool down and prepare for sleep.

Walking and Sleep Disorders

In addition to insomnia, there are other sleep disorders that can interfere with your ability to get a good night's sleep. Walking can be a helpful tool for managing conditions such as sleep apnea and restless legs syndrome (RLS), which are common causes of sleep disturbances.

- **Sleep Apnea**: Sleep apnea is a condition in which breathing repeatedly stops and starts during sleep, leading to fragmented sleep and daytime fatigue. Walking can help reduce the severity of sleep apnea by promoting weight loss and improving cardiovascular health. Excess weight, particularly around the neck, is a major risk factor for sleep apnea, and regular walking can help reduce this risk by promoting fat loss and improving overall fitness.

- **Restless Legs Syndrome (RLS)**: RLS is characterized by an uncontrollable urge to move the legs, particularly in the evening or during periods of rest. This can make it difficult to fall asleep or stay asleep. Walking helps alleviate the symptoms of RLS by improving circulation, reducing muscle tension, and providing an outlet for physical energy. Regular walking has been shown to reduce the frequency and severity of RLS symptoms, allowing for better sleep.

Maximizing the Sleep Benefits of Walking

To fully experience the sleep-enhancing benefits of walking, it's important to integrate walking into your daily routine in a way that supports your overall sleep hygiene. Here are some practical tips to help you get the most out of your walking routine for better sleep:

1. **Create a Consistent Walking Routine**
   Consistency is key when it comes to improving sleep. Aim to walk at the same time each day, whether it's in the morning, during lunch, or in the evening. Establishing a regular walking routine helps regulate your circadian rhythm, making it easier for your body to know when it's time to sleep.

2. **Focus on Relaxation**
   While brisk walking has its benefits, a slower, more relaxed pace may be better for promoting restful sleep, especially if you walk in the evening. Focus on breathing deeply, staying mindful of your surroundings, and letting go of any tension in your body as you walk.

3. **Pair Walking with a Calming Bedtime Routine**
    In addition to walking, create a calming bedtime routine that helps
    your body wind down for sleep. This could include activities like
    reading, taking a warm bath, or practicing relaxation techniques
    like deep breathing or meditation. Avoid stimulating activities like
    watching TV or using electronic devices, as these can interfere
    with your ability to fall asleep.

4. **Track Your Sleep Patterns**
    Consider using a sleep tracking app or device to monitor your
    sleep patterns as you incorporate walking into your routine.
    Tracking your sleep can provide insights into how your walking
    routine is affecting your rest and help you make any necessary
    adjustments.

5. **Stay Hydrated, But Not Too Late**
    Hydration is important for overall health, but drinking too much
    water right before bed can lead to frequent trips to the bathroom
    during the night. Make sure to drink plenty of water during the
    day, especially during and after your walks, but try to limit fluids
    in the hour or two before bedtime.

The Long-Term Sleep Benefits of Walking

Walking regularly offers long-term benefits for both your sleep quality
and overall health. As you continue to walk consistently, you'll likely
notice that falling asleep becomes easier, your sleep is less interrupted,
and you wake up feeling more energized. Over time, regular walking
helps establish a healthy sleep pattern, reducing the risk of sleep
disturbances and improving your quality of life.

Walking also supports other factors that contribute to better sleep, such as weight management, stress reduction, and cardiovascular health. By improving these areas, you'll not only sleep better but also feel better physically and mentally.

Conclusion: Walking for Restful, Restorative Sleep

Walking 4 miles a day is a natural and effective way to improve sleep quality, reduce insomnia, and wake up feeling refreshed and energized. By incorporating regular walking into your daily routine, you can support your body's natural sleep-wake cycle, reduce stress, and create the physical fatigue necessary for deep, restorative sleep.

Chapter 15: Stronger Bones and Joints – Walking for Bone Health and Mobility

As we age, maintaining strong bones and flexible joints becomes increasingly important for staying active, independent, and pain-free. Walking 4 miles a day is one of the best ways to support bone health and improve joint mobility. It is a low-impact, weight-bearing exercise that helps strengthen bones, keep joints lubricated, and reduce the risk of osteoporosis and arthritis-related complications.

In this chapter, we'll explore how walking helps strengthen bones, why it's essential for joint health, and how it can enhance mobility and flexibility as you age. You'll also learn practical tips for protecting your bones and joints while walking, especially if you're managing joint pain or arthritis.

The Importance of Bone Health

Bone health is crucial for maintaining a strong skeletal system, which supports your body and protects your organs. Bones are living tissues that constantly break down and rebuild themselves in a process known as remodeling. As you age, this balance can shift, and your bones may break down faster than they can rebuild, leading to bone loss and conditions like osteoporosis.

Osteoporosis is a condition where bones become weak, brittle, and more prone to fractures. It's often called the "silent disease" because it progresses without symptoms until a bone fracture occurs. Walking is one of the most effective ways to prevent or slow the progression of osteoporosis and maintain bone density as you age.

How Walking Strengthens Bones

Walking is a weight-bearing exercise, meaning it forces your bones to work against gravity. This type of exercise is essential for stimulating bone growth and maintaining bone density. When you walk, the stress on your bones triggers bone-forming cells called osteoblasts to build new bone tissue, making your bones stronger and more resilient over time.

Here's how walking helps improve bone health:

- **Building Bone Density**: Walking regularly helps preserve bone density by stimulating the production of new bone tissue. This is especially important as you age, as bone density naturally declines over time. By consistently walking 4 miles a day, you can slow bone loss and reduce the risk of fractures and osteoporosis.

- **Supporting Weight Loss**: Maintaining a healthy weight is important for bone health, as excess weight puts additional stress on your bones and joints. Walking helps you manage your weight, reducing the strain on your skeletal system and lowering the risk of bone-related issues.

- **Improving Circulation**: Walking improves blood flow to your bones, ensuring that they receive the nutrients and oxygen needed to stay healthy. Better circulation helps bones regenerate and repair themselves more efficiently, reducing the risk of bone-related complications.

- **Preventing Bone Loss**: For postmenopausal women and older adults, bone loss can be a significant concern. Walking can help prevent bone loss by slowing down the rate at which bones break down, allowing your body to maintain healthier, stronger bones for longer.

The Role of Walking in Joint Health

While walking is excellent for bone strength, it's also one of the best exercises for maintaining joint health and mobility. Unlike high-impact exercises that can put strain on your joints, walking is gentle and helps keep joints lubricated, flexible, and pain-free.

Here's how walking supports joint health:

- **Lubricating Joints**: Walking helps circulate synovial fluid, the natural lubricant found in your joints. This fluid reduces friction between your bones and allows for smoother movement. Keeping your joints well-lubricated helps prevent stiffness and reduces the risk of joint pain or injury, especially as you age.

- **Strengthening Supporting Muscles**: Walking engages the muscles surrounding your joints, particularly in the legs, hips, and lower back. Stronger muscles provide better support for your joints, reducing the pressure on them and helping to prevent wear and tear over time. This is particularly important for individuals with arthritis or joint pain, as walking helps stabilize the joints and alleviate discomfort.

- **Maintaining Range of Motion**: Walking moves your joints through their full range of motion, keeping them flexible and reducing stiffness. Regular movement helps preserve joint mobility, making it easier to perform everyday tasks like bending, reaching, or climbing stairs.

- **Reducing Inflammation**: Walking has anti-inflammatory effects that can help reduce joint inflammation, a key factor in conditions like arthritis. By improving circulation and reducing the production of inflammatory markers, walking helps manage joint pain and stiffness, allowing for greater comfort and mobility.

Walking for Arthritis Relief

For people with arthritis, joint pain and stiffness can make it challenging to stay active. However, walking is one of the best forms of exercise for managing arthritis symptoms and improving joint function. In fact, regular walking can help alleviate arthritis pain, increase joint flexibility, and reduce inflammation.

Here's why walking is beneficial for individuals with arthritis:

- **Reducing Pain**: Walking helps reduce arthritis-related pain by improving blood flow to the joints and promoting the release of endorphins, the body's natural painkillers. These endorphins help relieve discomfort and improve your overall sense of well-being.

- **Improving Joint Flexibility**: Regular walking helps keep your joints moving and flexible. This is especially important for people with arthritis, as inactivity can lead to further joint stiffness and reduced mobility. By walking daily, you can maintain or even improve your joint range of motion.

- **Strengthening the Muscles Around Joints**: Walking strengthens the muscles that support your joints, particularly in the knees, hips, and ankles. Stronger muscles help take pressure off the joints, reducing the risk of further damage and easing pain during movement.

- **Low-Impact, Joint-Friendly**: Walking is a low-impact exercise, meaning it doesn't place excessive stress on your joints. This makes it a safe and effective way to stay active without exacerbating arthritis symptoms. Start with short walks and gradually increase your distance and pace as your joints become more accustomed to regular movement.

Improving Mobility and Balance with Walking

One of the greatest challenges people face as they age is maintaining mobility and preventing falls. Walking not only helps strengthen your bones and joints but also improves your balance, coordination, and overall mobility, reducing the risk of falls and injuries.

Here's how walking enhances mobility and balance:

- **Strengthening Core and Lower Body Muscles**: Walking engages the muscles in your core, legs, and hips, which are essential for maintaining balance and stability. Stronger muscles help you stay steady on your feet, reducing the risk of trips or falls.

- **Improving Coordination**: Walking requires coordination between your muscles, joints, and nervous system. As you walk, your body constantly adjusts to changes in terrain, speed, and direction, which helps improve your overall coordination. Better coordination makes it easier to navigate your environment, especially in challenging conditions like uneven surfaces or stairs.

- **Enhancing Proprioception**: Proprioception is your body's ability to sense its position in space. Walking helps improve proprioception by making your body more aware of its movements and surroundings. This heightened sense of body awareness helps you react quickly to potential hazards, further reducing the risk of falls.

- **Maintaining Independence**: Regular walking helps preserve mobility and independence as you age. By staying active and maintaining joint flexibility, you'll be better equipped to perform daily activities like walking up stairs, bending down, or carrying groceries, allowing you to live more independently for longer.

Protecting Your Bones and Joints While Walking

While walking is one of the safest and most effective exercises for bone and joint health, it's important to take certain precautions to protect your body and prevent injury, especially if you have arthritis or other joint conditions. Here are some tips for protecting your bones and joints while walking:

1. **Wear Proper Footwear**
   Wearing supportive shoes is essential for protecting your joints while walking. Choose walking shoes that provide cushioning and arch support to absorb shock and reduce the impact on your feet, knees, and hips. Shoes with a wide toe box and good traction can also help prevent slips and falls.

2. **Warm Up and Cool Down**
   Before you start walking, take a few minutes to warm up your muscles and joints with gentle stretches or slow-paced walking. This helps increase blood flow and prepares your body for movement. After your walk, cool down with more stretches to improve flexibility and reduce muscle stiffness.

3. **Pace Yourself**

If you're new to walking or have joint pain, start slowly and gradually increase your distance and pace over time. Pushing yourself too hard can lead to injury or exacerbate joint pain. Listen to your body and take breaks when needed, especially if you feel any discomfort in your joints.

4. **Walk on Softer Surfaces**

Whenever possible, choose softer walking surfaces like dirt trails, grass, or rubberized tracks, which are easier on your joints compared to hard surfaces like concrete or asphalt. If you're walking on a treadmill, use the incline feature to reduce the impact on your knees and hips.

5. **Use Proper Posture**

Maintaining good posture while walking is essential for protecting your bones and joints. Keep your head up, shoulders relaxed, and core engaged. Avoid slouching or leaning forward, as this can strain your back and hips. Walking with good posture helps distribute your weight evenly across your joints, reducing the risk of discomfort or injury.

The Long-Term Benefits of Walking for Bone Health and Mobility

The benefits of walking for bone health and mobility go far beyond short-term relief. Walking regularly can help protect your bones and joints as you age, allowing you to maintain an active, independent lifestyle well into your later years. By strengthening your muscles, improving your balance, and preserving bone density, walking reduces the risk of falls, fractures, and joint deterioration.

For individuals with arthritis or osteoporosis, walking provides a gentle, effective way to manage symptoms and improve overall joint function. The more you walk, the stronger your bones and joints will become, reducing the likelihood of mobility issues as you age.

Conclusion: Walking for Strong Bones and Mobile Joints

Walking 4 miles a day is one of the most effective and sustainable ways to support bone health and improve joint mobility. Whether you're looking to prevent osteoporosis, manage arthritis symptoms, or simply maintain your independence as you age, walking offers a low-impact, weight-bearing solution that strengthens bones, lubricates joints, and enhances overall mobility.

Chapter 16: Immune System Support – Walking for a Stronger Immune Response

A healthy immune system is essential for protecting your body from illness, infection, and disease. While many factors influence immune function, regular physical activity, such as walking, plays a key role in keeping your immune system strong and resilient. Walking 4 miles a day not only helps you maintain overall health, but it also boosts your body's natural defenses, making you less susceptible to common illnesses like colds, the flu, and even more serious conditions.

In this chapter, we'll explore the science behind how walking strengthens your immune system, why it's effective in reducing the risk of illness, and how you can use walking as a natural way to support your body's defenses.

How the Immune System Works

Your immune system is a complex network of cells, tissues, and organs that work together to protect your body from harmful pathogens like bacteria, viruses, and fungi. It's made up of two main components:

- **Innate Immunity**: This is your body's first line of defense. It responds quickly to invaders by creating barriers (such as skin and mucous membranes) and deploying immune cells like white blood cells to destroy harmful organisms. This system provides general protection against a wide range of pathogens.

- **Adaptive Immunity**: This part of the immune system is more specialized and involves the production of antibodies that target specific pathogens. Once your body encounters a particular virus or bacteria, it "remembers" it, allowing your immune system to respond more effectively if you're exposed again in the future.

Maintaining a healthy immune system is crucial for preventing illness and ensuring that your body can respond effectively to threats. Walking helps enhance both innate and adaptive immunity, keeping your defenses strong.

How Walking Boosts the Immune System

Walking is one of the best ways to support immune function because it stimulates a wide range of processes that keep your body's defenses operating at their best. Here's how walking helps strengthen your immune system:

- **Increasing Circulation of Immune Cells**: Walking increases blood flow, which in turn enhances the circulation of immune cells like white blood cells (leukocytes) and lymphocytes. These cells are responsible for detecting and attacking harmful pathogens in your body. The increased circulation allows immune cells to move more efficiently throughout your system, making it easier for them to identify and eliminate threats.

- **Reducing Inflammation**: Chronic inflammation can weaken your immune system and make you more vulnerable to illness. Walking helps reduce inflammation by promoting the release of anti-inflammatory molecules and improving circulation. By reducing inflammation, your immune system is better equipped to respond to infections and heal the body.

- **Lowering Stress Levels**: Stress is a major factor that can suppress immune function, making it harder for your body to fight off illness. Walking helps lower stress by reducing cortisol levels and promoting the release of endorphins, which are natural mood enhancers. By managing stress effectively, you reduce its negative impact on your immune system, allowing it to function more efficiently.

- **Supporting Lymphatic Drainage**: The lymphatic system is an important part of your immune system, responsible for removing waste, toxins, and pathogens from your body. Unlike the circulatory system, the lymphatic system doesn't have a pump to move fluid; instead, it relies on muscle movement to keep lymph fluid circulating. Walking helps stimulate this movement, promoting better lymphatic drainage and ensuring that your immune system can filter out harmful substances more effectively.

The Relationship Between Exercise and Immune Function

Research consistently shows that moderate physical activity, such as walking, enhances immune function and reduces the risk of illness. While intense or prolonged exercise can sometimes suppress the immune system (especially if the body is overexerted), moderate exercise like walking strengthens it, making your body more resilient.

Here's why moderate exercise is so effective at boosting immunity:

- **Moderation is Key**: Moderate exercise helps regulate immune function by balancing the production of immune cells. It enhances the activity of key immune components like natural killer (NK) cells, which are responsible for identifying and attacking viruses and cancer cells. In contrast, overly intense exercise can cause a temporary suppression of immune function, leaving you more susceptible to infections. Walking strikes the perfect balance, providing enough stimulation to strengthen the immune system without overtaxing it.

- **Enhanced Immune Surveillance**: Walking increases immune surveillance, which refers to the immune system's ability to detect and respond to pathogens before they cause harm. Regular physical activity helps "train" your immune system to respond more effectively, improving your body's ability to ward off infections and illnesses.

- **Short and Long-Term Benefits**: Walking has both immediate and long-term benefits for immune function. After a single walk, immune cells circulate more efficiently, providing immediate protection against pathogens. Over time, regular walking strengthens your immune system, reducing the overall risk of developing chronic illnesses.

Walking to Prevent Common Illnesses

One of the most practical benefits of walking is its ability to reduce your risk of common illnesses like colds, the flu, and respiratory infections. Here's how walking helps protect you from everyday illnesses:

- **Cold and Flu Prevention**: Research has shown that people who engage in regular physical activity, including walking, are less likely to catch colds or the flu. A study published in the *American Journal of Medicine* found that people who walked briskly for 30 to 45 minutes a day experienced a 40-50% reduction in the number of sick days compared to sedentary individuals. Even if they did catch a cold, their symptoms were milder, and recovery was faster.

- **Respiratory Health**: Walking helps improve lung function and respiratory health, reducing the risk of respiratory infections. By increasing oxygen intake and improving circulation, walking ensures that your lungs stay healthy and better equipped to fend off infections. This is especially important during flu season or times when respiratory viruses are prevalent.

- **Supporting Gut Health**: Gut health is closely linked to immune function, as the gut is home to a large portion of your immune system. Walking promotes healthy digestion, reduces inflammation, and supports the growth of beneficial bacteria in the gut, all of which contribute to stronger immune defenses.

Walking for Long-Term Immune Health

While walking provides immediate immune benefits, it also plays a key role in maintaining long-term immune health. Regular walking can help protect you from more serious health conditions that weaken the immune system, such as chronic diseases and age-related decline.

Here's how walking supports immune health over the long term:

- **Reducing the Risk of Chronic Disease**: Chronic conditions like diabetes, heart disease, and obesity can weaken the immune system, making it harder for your body to fight infections. Walking helps reduce the risk of developing these diseases by promoting weight management, improving cardiovascular health, and regulating blood sugar levels. By staying active and healthy, you give your immune system a better chance to stay strong and function effectively.

- **Supporting Healthy Aging**: As we age, our immune systems naturally become less efficient, a process known as immunosenescence. Walking helps slow down this process by maintaining physical fitness, reducing inflammation, and supporting overall health. Regular walking can help older adults maintain a more resilient immune system, reducing the risk of infections and chronic diseases that become more common with age.

- **Strengthening the Body's Response to Vaccines**: Regular physical activity, including walking, has been shown to enhance the effectiveness of vaccines. Walking improves the body's immune response to vaccines by boosting the production of antibodies, making vaccinations more effective at preventing illness.

Practical Tips for Boosting Immune Health with Walking

To maximize the immune-boosting benefits of walking, it's important to develop a routine that supports your overall health and well-being. Here are some practical tips for using walking as a tool to strengthen your immune system:

1. **Walk Outdoors When Possible**
   Walking outdoors exposes you to fresh air and natural sunlight, which supports immune health. Sunlight stimulates the production of vitamin D, an essential nutrient that plays a critical role in immune function. Spending time in nature also reduces stress, which further strengthens your body's defenses.

2. **Stay Consistent**
   Consistency is key to maintaining a strong immune system. Aim

to walk 4 miles a day, most days of the week, to keep your immune cells circulating and your body's defenses primed. Even on days when you can't complete a full walk, try to incorporate some form of movement to stay active.

3. **Hydrate and Fuel Your Body**
    Staying hydrated is important for immune health, as it helps maintain healthy mucous membranes and keeps your lymphatic system functioning properly. Drink plenty of water before, during, and after your walk to stay hydrated. Additionally, fuel your body with nutrient-dense foods that support immune function, such as fruits, vegetables, whole grains, and lean proteins.

4. **Get Enough Rest**
    While walking boosts your immune system, it's also important to balance physical activity with adequate rest. Sleep is essential for immune function, as your body repairs and regenerates during rest. Make sure you're getting enough sleep each night to support your overall health and maximize the immune benefits of walking.

5. **Listen to Your Body**
    While walking is beneficial for immune health, it's important not to overdo it, especially if you're feeling under the weather. If you're experiencing symptoms of illness, it's okay to take a rest day and allow your body time to recover. Gentle movement, such as a short, slow-paced walk, can help stimulate circulation without putting too much strain on your body.

The Long-Term Immune Benefits of Walking

Walking regularly provides both immediate and long-term benefits for immune health. In the short term, walking helps circulate immune cells, reduce stress, and prevent common illnesses like colds and respiratory infections. Over the long term, walking supports a healthy immune system by reducing the risk of chronic diseases, enhancing vaccine effectiveness, and promoting overall well-being.

By making walking a part of your daily routine, you'll not only strengthen your immune system but also improve your overall health, allowing you to live a more vibrant and illness-free life.

Conclusion: Walking for a Stronger Immune System

Walking 4 miles a day is one of the most effective ways to boost your immune system, protect yourself from illness, and maintain overall health. By improving circulation, reducing stress, and supporting your body's natural defenses, walking helps keep your immune system strong and ready to fight off infections.

Chapter 17: Cardiovascular Endurance – Walking for Stamina and Energy

Cardiovascular endurance is the foundation of physical fitness and overall well-being. It determines how efficiently your heart, lungs, and muscles work together to sustain physical activity over extended periods of time. Whether you're climbing stairs, running errands, or simply going about your daily routine, having good cardiovascular endurance allows you to perform these activities with ease and without feeling fatigued. Walking 4 miles a day is one of the best ways to improve cardiovascular endurance, boost your energy levels, and enhance your overall stamina.

In this chapter, we'll explore how walking strengthens your cardiovascular system, the long-term benefits of increased stamina, and how to incorporate strategies into your walking routine to further boost endurance and energy levels.

Understanding Cardiovascular Endurance

Cardiovascular endurance, also known as aerobic endurance, refers to the ability of your heart, lungs, and blood vessels to deliver oxygen to your muscles during sustained physical activity. The more efficient your cardiovascular system is, the longer you can maintain physical activity without feeling fatigued. This endurance is vital for everyday tasks as well as more intense forms of exercise, and it's a key indicator of overall fitness and health.

Here's how walking improves cardiovascular endurance:

- **Heart Health**: Walking strengthens the heart muscle, allowing it to pump blood more efficiently. This means that your heart doesn't have to work as hard to circulate oxygen-rich blood throughout your body, improving endurance and reducing the risk of cardiovascular disease.

- **Lung Function**: Walking improves lung capacity and function, allowing you to take in more oxygen and expel carbon dioxide more effectively. The more oxygen your lungs can supply to your muscles, the longer you can sustain physical activity without feeling winded.

- **Muscle Efficiency**: Walking trains your muscles to use oxygen more efficiently, allowing them to perform better during exercise. Over time, your muscles become more adept at using oxygen to generate energy, which improves stamina and reduces fatigue.

- **Blood Flow and Oxygen Delivery**: Walking increases circulation, ensuring that more oxygen and nutrients are delivered to your muscles and organs. This improved blood flow helps your body maintain physical activity for longer periods without tiring.

How Walking Improves Cardiovascular Endurance

Walking is a highly effective form of aerobic exercise that gradually builds your cardiovascular endurance over time. The key to improving stamina through walking is consistency and progressive overload—gradually increasing the intensity and duration of your walks to challenge your heart, lungs, and muscles.

Here's how walking 4 miles a day helps build cardiovascular endurance:

- **Gradual Heart Rate Elevation**: Walking elevates your heart rate to a moderate level, which helps train your cardiovascular system to handle increased demands. Over time, your heart becomes stronger and more efficient, allowing you to maintain physical activity for longer periods without feeling fatigued.

- **Improved VO2 Max**: VO2 max is a measure of the maximum amount of oxygen your body can use during exercise. Walking regularly helps increase your VO2 max, which means your body can utilize more oxygen during physical activity, improving stamina and energy levels. A higher VO2 max is associated with better cardiovascular health and overall fitness.

- **Increased Capillary Density**: Walking promotes the growth of new capillaries (tiny blood vessels) in your muscles. These capillaries deliver oxygen and nutrients to your muscles more efficiently, allowing them to sustain physical activity for longer periods. As capillary density increases, your muscles become better at performing aerobic exercises like walking.

- **Muscle Endurance**: Walking builds endurance in your leg muscles, particularly the calves, quadriceps, hamstrings, and glutes. As these muscles become stronger and more efficient, they can sustain movement for longer periods without fatigue. This increased muscle endurance translates to better overall stamina for daily activities.

The Benefits of Improved Cardiovascular Endurance

Improving your cardiovascular endurance through walking offers a wide range of benefits that go beyond fitness. Here are some of the most important advantages:

- **Increased Energy Levels**: One of the first benefits you'll notice as your endurance improves is a significant boost in energy levels. Walking enhances your body's ability to produce energy, allowing you to go through your day with less fatigue. You'll find it easier to perform tasks, whether it's going up stairs, carrying groceries, or playing with your kids, without getting winded.

- **Better Mental Clarity**: Cardiovascular exercise, like walking, increases blood flow to the brain, improving cognitive function and mental clarity. This enhanced brain function can help you stay more focused and alert throughout the day, reducing brain fog and boosting productivity.

- **Improved Recovery**: When your cardiovascular endurance is high, your body recovers more quickly from physical exertion. This means that after a walk or a workout, you'll experience less muscle soreness and fatigue, allowing you to get back to your routine more quickly.

- **Reduced Risk of Chronic Diseases**: Walking regularly helps reduce the risk of chronic conditions such as heart disease, diabetes, and stroke. Improved cardiovascular endurance leads to better heart health, lower blood pressure, and more stable blood sugar levels, all of which contribute to a longer, healthier life.

- **Enhanced Mood and Stress Relief**: Cardiovascular exercise like walking releases endorphins, which are natural mood boosters. Walking helps reduce stress, anxiety, and depression, improving your overall sense of well-being. The more consistent you are with walking, the more resilient you become to stress.

Walking Strategies to Boost Cardiovascular Endurance

To maximize the cardiovascular benefits of walking and continue improving your stamina, it's important to gradually increase the intensity and duration of your walks. Here are some strategies to help you boost your endurance:

1. **Increase Your Distance Gradually**
   If you're comfortable walking 4 miles a day, try gradually increasing your distance to challenge your cardiovascular system. Aim to add a half-mile or an extra 10-15 minutes to your walks each week. This progressive overload will help your heart, lungs, and muscles adapt to increased demands, improving endurance over time.

2. **Incorporate Interval Training**
   Interval training involves alternating between periods of brisk walking and slower-paced walking. This method elevates your heart rate during the fast intervals, challenging your cardiovascular system and improving stamina. For example, you can walk briskly for 2 minutes, followed by 1 minute of slower walking, and repeat this pattern throughout your walk.

3. **Walk on Different Terrains**
   Walking on varied terrains, such as hills, trails, or stairs, adds resistance and challenges your cardiovascular system to work harder. Walking uphill or on uneven surfaces engages more muscles, improves coordination, and increases calorie burn, all of which enhance endurance.

4. **Increase Your Walking Speed**
   To build cardiovascular endurance, focus on increasing your

walking speed. A brisk pace of 3 to 4 miles per hour is ideal for improving stamina. If you're comfortable with your current pace, try walking a little faster to challenge yourself. Power walking, which involves exaggerated arm movements and a faster stride, can also boost endurance.

5. **Use a Pedometer or Fitness Tracker**
   Tracking your steps, distance, and pace can help you stay motivated and measure your progress. Use a pedometer or fitness tracker to monitor your daily activity and set goals for improving your endurance. Aim to gradually increase the number of steps or the distance you cover each day to challenge your cardiovascular system.

Maintaining Cardiovascular Endurance Over Time

Building cardiovascular endurance through walking is an ongoing process, and consistency is key to maintaining the benefits. Here's how to ensure that you continue to improve and maintain your stamina over the long term:

- **Stay Consistent**: Make walking a regular part of your daily routine. Aim to walk at least 4 miles a day, most days of the week, to maintain your cardiovascular fitness and continue improving your endurance. Consistency is key to sustaining the benefits of walking and ensuring that your stamina doesn't decline.

- **Challenge Yourself**: As your cardiovascular endurance improves, continue to challenge yourself by increasing the intensity or duration of your walks. This could mean walking at a faster pace, incorporating hills or intervals, or extending your daily distance. Keeping your routine fresh and challenging prevents plateaus and ensures that you continue making progress.

- **Incorporate Strength Training**: While walking is excellent for cardiovascular endurance, adding strength training to your routine can further improve your stamina and overall fitness. Stronger muscles support your cardiovascular system by helping you perform physical activities with less effort. Consider adding bodyweight exercises like squats, lunges, and push-ups to your routine to enhance your endurance.

- **Rest and Recover**: While consistency is important, so is rest. Make sure to listen to your body and allow time for recovery when needed. Rest days give your muscles and cardiovascular system a chance to recover and rebuild, preventing burnout and overtraining.

The Long-Term Benefits of Cardiovascular Endurance

The long-term benefits of improving your cardiovascular endurance through walking extend far beyond just fitness. A strong cardiovascular system supports every aspect of your health, from reducing the risk of chronic diseases to improving mental clarity, energy levels, and emotional well-being.

As you continue walking regularly, you'll notice that daily activities become easier, your energy levels remain high throughout the day, and your overall physical and mental resilience improves. Whether you're looking to enhance your athletic performance, improve your quality of life, or simply stay healthy as you age, walking for cardiovascular endurance is one of the most effective ways to achieve these goals.

Conclusion: Walking for Stamina and Energy

Walking 4 miles a day is one of the best ways to build and maintain cardiovascular endurance, allowing you to enjoy higher energy levels, improved stamina, and better overall health. By challenging your cardiovascular system with regular, consistent walking, you'll experience increased endurance, reduced fatigue, and a greater ability to perform everyday tasks with ease.

Chapter 18: Digestive Health – Walking for a Balanced Gut and Better Digestion

Your digestive system plays a crucial role in your overall health, breaking down food into nutrients your body needs and eliminating waste. A healthy digestive system not only supports nutrient absorption but also affects your energy levels, immune function, and even mental well-being. Walking 4 miles a day can have a profound impact on your digestive health by improving digestion, preventing digestive disorders, and promoting a balanced gut microbiome.

In this chapter, we'll explore how walking supports digestive function, why it's beneficial for gut health, and how to incorporate walking into your routine to enhance digestion and prevent common digestive issues.

The Digestive System: How It Works

The digestive system is a complex network of organs that work together to break down food into nutrients, absorb those nutrients into the bloodstream, and eliminate waste. It includes the mouth, esophagus, stomach, intestines, and colon, as well as accessory organs like the liver, pancreas, and gallbladder.

Here's a brief overview of the digestive process:

- **Mouth**: Digestion begins in the mouth, where chewing and saliva start breaking down food.
- **Stomach**: Food moves to the stomach, where it's mixed with stomach acid and digestive enzymes that break it down further.
- **Small Intestine**: Most nutrient absorption occurs in the small intestine, where food is broken down into its smallest components—carbohydrates, proteins, and fats.
- **Large Intestine**: The large intestine absorbs water and minerals while forming waste into stool for elimination.

A healthy digestive system is essential for ensuring that your body gets the nutrients it needs to function properly. Walking is one of the simplest ways to support your digestive system, helping it work efficiently and promoting overall gut health.

How Walking Improves Digestion

Walking offers a wide range of benefits for your digestive system, from enhancing digestion and nutrient absorption to preventing constipation and reducing bloating. Here's how walking helps improve digestive function:

- **Promoting Regular Bowel Movements**: Walking stimulates the muscles in your digestive tract, helping food move through your intestines more efficiently. This increased movement, known as gastrointestinal motility, helps prevent constipation and ensures that waste is eliminated regularly. Regular bowel movements are essential for maintaining digestive health and preventing discomfort.

- **Reducing Bloating and Gas**: Bloating and gas are common digestive issues that can cause discomfort and embarrassment. Walking helps relieve these symptoms by promoting the movement of gas through the intestines and preventing the buildup of air in the digestive tract. The gentle movement of walking encourages your body to release trapped gas, reducing bloating and promoting a flatter stomach.

- **Speeding Up Digestion**: Walking after meals can help speed up digestion by stimulating the production of digestive enzymes and increasing blood flow to the digestive organs. This helps your body break down food more quickly and absorb nutrients more efficiently, preventing feelings of sluggishness or heaviness after eating.

- **Supporting Peristalsis**: Peristalsis is the wave-like muscle contractions that move food through your digestive system. Walking enhances peristalsis by stimulating the muscles in your intestines, helping food move smoothly through the digestive tract. This reduces the risk of digestive issues like indigestion, acid reflux, and constipation.

- **Reducing the Risk of Digestive Disorders**: Regular physical activity, such as walking, helps reduce the risk of developing digestive disorders like irritable bowel syndrome (IBS) and gastroesophageal reflux disease (GERD). By improving digestion and preventing constipation, walking helps maintain a healthy gut and reduces the risk of inflammation or irritation in the digestive tract.

Walking for Gut Health

In addition to supporting digestion, walking has a positive impact on gut health by promoting a balanced microbiome. The gut microbiome is a community of trillions of bacteria, viruses, and fungi that live in your digestive tract. A healthy, diverse microbiome is essential for good digestion, immune function, and overall health.

Here's how walking supports a healthy gut microbiome:

- **Reducing Inflammation**: Chronic inflammation can disrupt the balance of bacteria in your gut, leading to digestive issues and other health problems. Walking helps reduce inflammation throughout the body, including the gut. By lowering levels of inflammatory markers, walking promotes a healthier, more balanced microbiome.

- **Promoting Gut Motility**: Walking improves the movement of food and waste through the digestive system, which helps maintain the balance of bacteria in your gut. When food moves too slowly through the intestines, it can lead to an overgrowth of harmful bacteria, contributing to bloating, gas, and other digestive issues. Walking helps maintain gut motility, supporting the growth of beneficial bacteria.

- **Improving Stress Management**: Stress is closely linked to gut health, as the gut and brain communicate through the gut-brain axis. High levels of stress can disrupt the balance of bacteria in your gut, leading to digestive problems like IBS. Walking helps reduce stress by lowering cortisol levels and promoting relaxation, which in turn supports a healthier gut.

- **Boosting Immune Function**: Your gut plays a key role in your immune system, and walking enhances immune function by supporting the gut's ability to fend off harmful pathogens. A healthy gut microbiome strengthens your immune system, making it easier for your body to fight infections and maintain overall health.

The Best Time to Walk for Digestive Health

To get the most digestive benefits from walking, it's helpful to time your walks around meals. Here are some guidelines for when to walk to optimize digestion:

- **After Meals**: Walking after meals is one of the best ways to support digestion. A post-meal walk helps stimulate the production of digestive enzymes and speeds up the digestive process, preventing feelings of heaviness or discomfort after eating. Even a short 10-15 minute walk after a meal can make a significant difference in how well your body digests food.

- **Morning Walks**: Walking in the morning, especially on an empty stomach, can help kickstart your digestive system and promote regular bowel movements. Morning walks also boost circulation and metabolism, helping your body process food more efficiently throughout the day.

- **Evening Walks**: If you experience bloating or digestive discomfort in the evening, a gentle walk after dinner can help relieve these symptoms. Walking in the evening helps prevent indigestion and acid reflux by encouraging food to move through your digestive tract, rather than allowing it to sit in your stomach.

Walking for Digestive Disorders

For people with digestive disorders like irritable bowel syndrome (IBS), gastroesophageal reflux disease (GERD), or chronic constipation, walking can be an effective way to manage symptoms and improve overall digestive health.

Here's how walking helps with specific digestive conditions:

- **Irritable Bowel Syndrome (IBS)**: IBS is a common digestive disorder that causes symptoms like abdominal pain, bloating, diarrhea, and constipation. Walking helps manage IBS symptoms by promoting regular bowel movements, reducing stress, and improving gut motility. Regular walking can help prevent IBS flare-ups and improve overall gut function.

- **Gastroesophageal Reflux Disease (GERD)**: GERD occurs when stomach acid flows back into the esophagus, causing heartburn and indigestion. Walking after meals can help prevent acid reflux by promoting the downward movement of food and acid in the stomach. However, it's important to avoid vigorous exercise immediately after eating, as this can exacerbate GERD symptoms. A gentle walk is ideal for managing GERD.

- **Chronic Constipation**: Walking is one of the most effective natural remedies for chronic constipation. By stimulating the muscles in the intestines, walking helps improve bowel motility and promotes regular, healthy bowel movements. Walking also helps soften stool by improving hydration and circulation, making it easier to pass.

Practical Tips for Walking to Improve Digestion

To get the most digestive benefits from walking, it's important to establish a routine that supports your gut health and overall well-being. Here are some practical tips for using walking to improve digestion:

1. **Walk After Meals**
   Incorporate a short walk after each meal to help your body digest food more efficiently. Aim for a gentle 10-15 minute walk after breakfast, lunch, and dinner to stimulate digestion and prevent bloating.

2. **Stay Hydrated**

Hydration is key to healthy digestion, as it helps move food through the digestive tract and prevents constipation. Drink plenty of water before, during, and after your walks to support your digestive system. Staying hydrated also helps your body absorb nutrients more effectively.

3. **Avoid Overeating**

Large meals can slow down digestion and cause discomfort, especially if you plan to walk afterward. To avoid this, eat smaller, more frequent meals throughout the day, and avoid overeating at any one sitting. This helps your digestive system process food more efficiently and prevents indigestion.

4. **Focus on Mindful Eating**

Mindful eating can enhance the digestive benefits of walking by helping you tune in to your body's hunger and fullness cues. When you eat mindfully, you're more likely to stop eating before you feel too full, which reduces the likelihood of digestive discomfort. Pair mindful eating with regular walking for optimal digestive health.

5. **Listen to Your Body**

Pay attention to how your body responds to walking and make adjustments as needed. If you experience digestive discomfort, try walking at a slower pace or shortening your walk. On the other hand, if you find that walking helps relieve symptoms, consider increasing the duration or frequency of your walks.

The Long-Term Digestive Benefits of Walking

The benefits of walking for digestive health extend far beyond immediate relief from bloating or constipation. Regular walking promotes long-term gut health by improving digestion, supporting a balanced microbiome, and reducing the risk of chronic digestive disorders.

By making walking a regular part of your routine, you'll not only improve your digestive function but also experience better energy levels, reduced stress, and enhanced overall well-being. A healthy gut is the foundation of good health, and walking is one of the most effective ways to support and maintain that foundation.

Conclusion: Walking for a Balanced Gut and Better Digestion

Walking 4 miles a day is a simple and effective way to improve digestion, promote a healthy gut microbiome, and prevent common digestive issues like bloating and constipation. By incorporating regular walks into your routine, you'll support your body's ability to process food efficiently, absorb nutrients, and eliminate waste.

Chapter 19: Mental Clarity – Walking for Focus, Memory, and Cognitive Function

In addition to its physical health benefits, walking has a profound impact on mental clarity, memory, and overall cognitive function. Whether you're struggling with brain fog, looking to boost productivity, or aiming to enhance memory and focus, walking can play a significant role in improving your mental performance. Research has consistently shown that regular physical activity, particularly walking, stimulates brain function, supports neuroplasticity, and enhances mental sharpness.

In this chapter, we'll explore how walking affects brain health, the ways in which it boosts cognitive function, and practical strategies for using walking as a tool to improve focus, memory, and overall mental clarity.

The Connection Between Walking and Brain Health

Your brain relies on oxygen and nutrients delivered by your blood to function at its best. Walking increases blood flow, delivering more oxygen and glucose to the brain, which are essential for cognitive function. The more active you are, the better your brain works, as walking stimulates processes that protect brain cells, improve neural connections, and even support the growth of new brain cells.

Here's how walking directly impacts brain health:

- **Increased Blood Flow to the Brain**: Walking increases heart rate and circulation, which leads to more oxygen and nutrients being delivered to the brain. This increased blood flow helps improve brain function, mental clarity, and cognitive performance.

- **Stimulating Neurogenesis**: Walking promotes neurogenesis, the process by which new neurons (brain cells) are created.

Neurogenesis plays a key role in memory and learning, and regular physical activity like walking supports the growth of new neurons, particularly in the hippocampus, the brain region responsible for memory.

- **Supporting Neuroplasticity**: Neuroplasticity refers to the brain's ability to reorganize itself by forming new neural connections. Walking enhances neuroplasticity, allowing your brain to adapt to new experiences, learn new skills, and recover from injuries or age-related cognitive decline. This is crucial for maintaining mental sharpness and cognitive resilience as you age.

- **Reducing Brain Inflammation**: Inflammation in the brain has been linked to cognitive decline and neurodegenerative diseases like Alzheimer's. Walking helps reduce inflammation in the body, including the brain, which protects against cognitive impairment and promotes long-term brain health.

How Walking Improves Mental Clarity and Focus

Walking is a powerful tool for improving mental clarity and focus. Whether you're dealing with brain fog or simply need a mental boost during a busy day, walking can help clear your mind, enhance concentration, and sharpen your cognitive abilities.

Here's how walking enhances focus and mental clarity:

- **Boosting Energy Levels**: One of the reasons people experience brain fog or mental fatigue is a lack of energy. Walking helps boost energy levels by increasing circulation and oxygen flow to the brain, making you feel more alert and focused. Even a short walk can revitalize your mind and improve your ability to concentrate on tasks.

- **Improving Attention and Concentration**: Walking increases the production of neurotransmitters like dopamine and norepinephrine, which are associated with attention and focus. These neurotransmitters help improve your ability to concentrate on tasks and stay mentally engaged for longer periods without distraction.

- **Enhancing Cognitive Flexibility**: Cognitive flexibility is the brain's ability to switch between different tasks or thought processes. Walking has been shown to improve cognitive flexibility by stimulating brain activity and promoting neuroplasticity. This makes it easier to shift focus, solve problems, and adapt to new challenges.

- **Reducing Mental Fatigue**: Mental fatigue occurs when your brain becomes overloaded with information or tasks, making it harder to focus. Walking helps reduce mental fatigue by giving your brain a break and allowing it to reset. The rhythmic motion of walking promotes relaxation and mental recovery, helping you return to tasks with a clearer, more focused mind.

Walking for Memory Enhancement

In addition to improving focus and clarity, walking plays a key role in enhancing memory. Regular walking has been linked to improved short-term and long-term memory, as well as a reduced risk of age-related memory decline.

Here's how walking supports memory function:

- **Strengthening the Hippocampus**: The hippocampus is the part of the brain responsible for memory and learning, and it's particularly sensitive to the effects of aging. Walking helps protect the hippocampus by promoting neurogenesis and increasing blood flow to this region, which strengthens its ability to store and retrieve information.

- **Improving Working Memory**: Working memory is the ability to hold and manipulate information in your mind for short periods of time. Walking has been shown to improve working memory by enhancing brain activity in regions responsible for information processing and retention.

- **Reducing Memory Decline**: As we age, it's common to experience some degree of memory decline. However, regular physical activity like walking can help slow this process by protecting brain cells and reducing inflammation. Studies have shown that older adults who walk regularly are less likely to experience memory loss and are more likely to maintain cognitive function as they age.

- **Stimulating the Release of BDNF**: Walking increases the production of brain-derived neurotrophic factor (BDNF), a protein that promotes the growth and survival of neurons. BDNF is essential for memory formation and learning, and higher levels of BDNF are associated with better memory and cognitive function.

Walking for Mental Health and Emotional Well-Being

In addition to its cognitive benefits, walking has a positive impact on mental health and emotional well-being. By reducing stress, anxiety, and depression, walking helps create a mental environment that is conducive to clarity, focus, and productivity.

Here's how walking improves mental health and emotional well-being:

- **Reducing Stress and Anxiety**: Walking helps lower cortisol levels, the hormone associated with stress. This reduction in cortisol promotes relaxation and mental calm, making it easier to focus and think clearly. Walking also stimulates the release of endorphins, which are natural mood enhancers that help alleviate feelings of anxiety and depression.

- **Improving Mood**: Walking has been shown to improve mood by increasing serotonin and dopamine levels in the brain. These neurotransmitters play a key role in regulating mood and emotional balance. A positive mood is essential for maintaining mental clarity and focus, as stress and negative emotions can interfere with cognitive performance.

- **Enhancing Creativity**: Walking is a well-known tool for boosting creativity. The rhythmic, repetitive motion of walking allows your mind to wander, encouraging new ideas and creative insights. Many people find that they come up with their best ideas while walking, as the act of walking promotes divergent thinking and mental relaxation.

Practical Tips for Using Walking to Boost Mental Clarity and Focus

To maximize the mental clarity and cognitive benefits of walking, it's important to incorporate walking into your daily routine in a way that supports your brain health and productivity. Here are some practical tips for using walking to boost focus, memory, and mental sharpness:

1. **Take Short Walking Breaks**

   If you're working or studying for extended periods, take short walking breaks to reset your mind and improve focus. Even a 10-minute walk can enhance your mental clarity and help you return to your tasks with renewed concentration. Aim to take a short walk every hour or two to keep your brain sharp and engaged.

2. **Walk Outdoors for Maximum Benefits**

   Walking outdoors in nature offers additional cognitive benefits beyond physical movement. Spending time in natural environments has been shown to reduce mental fatigue, improve mood, and enhance cognitive function. If possible, take your walks in a park, forest, or near water to experience the restorative effects of nature.

3. **Practice Mindful Walking**

   Mindful walking involves focusing on the present moment, paying attention to your surroundings, and observing your thoughts without judgment. This practice helps clear mental clutter and reduces distractions, improving your ability to focus and think clearly. During your walks, focus on your breath, the feeling of your feet hitting the ground, and the sights and sounds around you.

4. **Incorporate Walking into Problem-Solving**

   If you're stuck on a problem or need to think through a challenging situation, take a walk to clear your mind. Walking promotes creative thinking and mental flexibility, making it easier to come up with solutions and new ideas. Many people find that they are better able to solve problems after taking a break for a walk.

5. Walk in the Morning to Boost Mental Performance
Walking in the morning helps set a positive tone for the day and boosts mental clarity and focus. A morning walk increases circulation, oxygenates the brain, and enhances cognitive function, allowing you to start your day with improved mental sharpness and energy. If you have a busy or stressful day ahead, a morning walk can help you feel more prepared and mentally resilient.

The Long-Term Cognitive Benefits of Walking

Walking regularly offers long-term benefits for cognitive function, memory, and mental health. Over time, consistent walking helps protect against age-related cognitive decline, reduces the risk of neurodegenerative diseases, and promotes lifelong brain health. The more you walk, the more resilient your brain becomes to stress, aging, and cognitive challenges.

For older adults, walking is especially beneficial for maintaining cognitive function and reducing the risk of conditions like Alzheimer's disease and dementia. By enhancing neuroplasticity and promoting the growth of new brain cells, walking helps preserve mental sharpness and memory well into old age.

Conclusion: Walking for Focus, Memory, and Cognitive Function

Walking 4 miles a day is one of the most effective ways to improve mental clarity, enhance memory, and boost cognitive function. By increasing blood flow to the brain, promoting neurogenesis, and reducing mental fatigue, walking helps you stay focused, sharp, and mentally resilient throughout the day.

Chapter 20: Healthy Aging – Walking for Vitality and Independence

Aging is a natural part of life, but the way we age can greatly depend on our lifestyle choices. One of the most powerful tools for aging gracefully is walking. Regular physical activity, particularly walking, has been shown to slow the aging process, maintain physical and mental vitality, and help older adults remain independent longer. Walking not only supports physical health but also boosts mental and emotional well-being, making it one of the most effective ways to promote healthy aging.

In this chapter, we'll explore how walking supports healthy aging, how it helps maintain independence and mobility, and why it's so effective in reducing the risk of age-related diseases and conditions.

The Physical Benefits of Walking for Healthy Aging

As we age, our bodies undergo a series of changes, including a natural decline in muscle mass, bone density, and joint flexibility. These changes can lead to frailty, a higher risk of falls, and a reduction in mobility. However, walking can counteract many of these age-related changes by keeping the body strong, flexible, and functional.

Here's how walking supports physical health as you age:

- **Maintaining Muscle Mass**: Sarcopenia, or the age-related loss of muscle mass, is a common issue that can lead to weakness and reduced mobility. Walking engages the muscles in your legs, hips, and core, helping to preserve muscle mass and strength. Regular walking also enhances muscle endurance, allowing you to stay active and independent for longer.

- **Improving Bone Density**: Walking is a weight-bearing exercise, meaning it helps stimulate bone growth and maintain bone density. This is especially important for older adults, as bone density naturally decreases with age, leading to conditions like osteoporosis. Walking helps slow the progression of bone loss, reducing the risk of fractures and promoting strong, healthy bones.

- **Supporting Joint Flexibility**: Aging often leads to stiffness in the joints, which can make movement more difficult and increase the risk of injury. Walking helps keep your joints lubricated and flexible, improving range of motion and reducing joint pain. Regular movement is key to maintaining joint health and preventing conditions like arthritis from limiting your mobility.

- **Enhancing Cardiovascular Health**: Walking strengthens the heart and improves circulation, helping to lower blood pressure, reduce cholesterol levels, and protect against heart disease. Cardiovascular health is crucial for aging well, as a strong heart ensures that your body can continue to function efficiently as you age.

- **Maintaining a Healthy Weight**: Maintaining a healthy weight is essential for reducing the strain on your joints, improving mobility, and preventing chronic diseases. Walking helps burn calories, promote fat loss, and support a healthy metabolism, making it easier to maintain a healthy body weight as you age.

Walking for Mobility and Independence

One of the greatest fears many people have about aging is losing their independence. As mobility declines, simple tasks like walking up stairs, carrying groceries, or even getting out of bed can become challenging. However, walking is one of the most effective ways to preserve mobility and maintain independence well into old age.

Here's how walking supports mobility and independence:

- **Strengthening Lower Body Muscles**: Walking engages the muscles in your legs, hips, and glutes, which are essential for balance and mobility. Strong lower body muscles help you perform daily activities like standing up from a chair, climbing stairs, and walking without assistance. Regular walking helps maintain this strength, reducing the risk of falls and improving your ability to move independently.

- **Improving Balance and Coordination**: As we age, our balance and coordination naturally decline, increasing the risk of falls and injuries. Walking helps improve balance by engaging stabilizing muscles and promoting proprioception (the body's sense of its position in space). Better balance reduces the risk of falls, which are a leading cause of injury in older adults.

- **Reducing the Risk of Falls**: Falls are a major concern for older adults, often leading to fractures, hospitalizations, and a loss of independence. Walking helps reduce the risk of falls by strengthening muscles, improving balance, and increasing flexibility. By staying active, you'll be better equipped to prevent falls and maintain your independence.

- **Maintaining Functional Mobility**: Functional mobility refers to your ability to perform daily tasks that require movement, such as getting dressed, cooking, or walking around your home. Walking enhances functional mobility by keeping your muscles and joints in good working order, allowing you to remain self-sufficient and perform everyday tasks without assistance.

Mental and Emotional Benefits of Walking for Aging

In addition to its physical benefits, walking has a profound impact on mental and emotional well-being as we age. Cognitive decline, depression, and social isolation are common issues faced by older adults, but walking can help mitigate these challenges by supporting brain health and promoting emotional resilience.

Here's how walking benefits mental and emotional well-being in older adults:

- **Preserving Cognitive Function**: Cognitive decline is a major concern for many people as they age, but walking can help protect brain health and reduce the risk of conditions like dementia and Alzheimer's disease. Walking increases blood flow to the brain, supports neuroplasticity, and promotes the growth of new brain cells, all of which help preserve memory, attention, and cognitive function.

- **Reducing the Risk of Dementia**: Regular physical activity, including walking, has been shown to reduce the risk of developing dementia by improving cardiovascular health, reducing inflammation, and supporting brain function. Studies have found that older adults who walk regularly are less likely to develop dementia and more likely to maintain cognitive function into old age.

- **Boosting Mood and Reducing Depression**: Depression and anxiety are common among older adults, especially those who experience social isolation or chronic health conditions. Walking helps boost mood by stimulating the release of endorphins, which are natural mood enhancers. Regular walking can also reduce feelings of loneliness by encouraging social interaction, especially if you walk with friends or join a walking group.

- **Enhancing Quality of Life**: Walking promotes a sense of independence, purpose, and well-being, all of which are important for maintaining a high quality of life as you age. By staying active and engaged with the world around you, walking helps you maintain a positive outlook and a greater sense of control over your life.

Walking to Prevent Age-Related Diseases

As we age, the risk of developing chronic diseases like heart disease, diabetes, and arthritis increases. However, walking has been shown to reduce the risk of many age-related diseases, helping you stay healthy and active well into old age.

Here's how walking helps prevent common age-related conditions:

- **Reducing the Risk of Heart Disease**: Heart disease is the leading cause of death in older adults, but walking can significantly reduce the risk by improving cardiovascular health. Walking helps lower blood pressure, reduce cholesterol, and improve circulation, all of which protect the heart and reduce the likelihood of heart attacks and strokes.

- **Preventing Type 2 Diabetes**: Walking helps regulate blood sugar levels and improves insulin sensitivity, reducing the risk of developing type 2 diabetes. For those who already have diabetes, walking can help manage the condition by promoting better blood sugar control and reducing the need for medication.

- **Managing Arthritis Symptoms**: Arthritis is a common condition that causes joint pain and stiffness, but regular walking can help manage symptoms by keeping joints flexible and reducing inflammation. Walking also strengthens the muscles around your joints, providing better support and reducing the strain on your joints during movement.

- **Supporting Respiratory Health**: Walking improves lung function and increases oxygen intake, helping to maintain respiratory health as you age. Regular walking can reduce the risk of respiratory infections and conditions like chronic obstructive pulmonary disease (COPD), allowing you to breathe easier and stay active.

Practical Tips for Walking to Promote Healthy Aging

To maximize the benefits of walking for healthy aging, it's important to make walking a regular part of your routine. Here are some practical tips for using walking to support vitality and independence as you age:

1. **Start Slow and Build Up Gradually**
   If you're new to walking or haven't been physically active in a while, start with short, slow walks and gradually increase your distance and pace over time. Aim to walk for at least 30 minutes a day, most days of the week, to improve your overall health and fitness.

2. **Incorporate Strength Training**
   To enhance the muscle-building benefits of walking, consider

adding light strength training exercises to your routine. Strengthening your muscles helps improve balance and mobility, making walking more effective for maintaining independence. Bodyweight exercises like squats, lunges, and calf raises can be easily incorporated into your walking routine.

3.   **Wear Supportive Footwear**
Wearing comfortable, supportive shoes is essential for preventing foot and joint pain while walking. Choose shoes with good cushioning and arch support to reduce the impact on your knees, hips, and lower back. If necessary, consider using orthotics for added support.

4.   **Use Walking Poles for Stability**
If balance is a concern, consider using walking poles to provide extra stability and reduce the risk of falls. Walking poles help engage your upper body muscles, improve posture, and provide additional support for your joints, making walking safer and more comfortable.

5.   **Make Walking Social**
Walking with friends, family, or a walking group can make the activity more enjoyable and help prevent feelings of isolation. Social interaction is important for mental health and emotional well-being, and walking with others provides an opportunity to stay connected and engaged with your community.

The Long-Term Benefits of Walking for Aging Well

The long-term benefits of walking for healthy aging extend far beyond physical fitness. Regular walking helps preserve mobility, independence, and cognitive function, allowing you to enjoy a higher quality of life as you age. By reducing the risk of chronic diseases, improving mental health, and supporting physical vitality, walking ensures that you can stay active, engaged, and independent for as long as possible.

As you continue walking for better health, you'll experience the ongoing benefits of improved strength, balance, and mental sharpness, all of which are essential for aging gracefully.

Conclusion: Walking for Vitality and Independence

Walking 4 miles a day is one of the most effective ways to promote healthy aging, maintain physical vitality, and preserve independence as you grow older. By supporting cardiovascular health, strengthening muscles and bones, and improving cognitive function, walking helps you age with strength, confidence, and resilience.

Chapter 21: Emotional Resilience – Walking for Mental Strength and Positivity

Emotional resilience is the ability to cope with life's challenges, stressors, and setbacks while maintaining a positive outlook. In a world filled with uncertainties, having emotional resilience is key to mental health and well-being. Walking 4 miles a day is not only a powerful tool for physical fitness, but it also significantly contributes to building emotional resilience. The act of walking provides a healthy outlet for stress, enhances your mood, and fosters mental clarity, all of which help you stay mentally strong in the face of adversity.

In this chapter, we'll explore how walking boosts emotional resilience, how it helps you manage stress and anxiety, and practical strategies for using walking to cultivate mental strength and a positive mindset.

Understanding Emotional Resilience

Emotional resilience is the mental toughness that allows you to bounce back from adversity, whether it's a stressful job, personal challenges, or unexpected life changes. Resilience doesn't mean avoiding stress or negative emotions, but rather developing the capacity to recover quickly and maintain your well-being despite these challenges.

The good news is that emotional resilience can be cultivated, and one of the most effective ways to do so is through physical activity. Walking offers a practical, accessible way to build mental and emotional strength, equipping you with the tools you need to handle stress, regulate emotions, and maintain a positive outlook.

How Walking Builds Emotional Resilience

Walking plays a crucial role in building emotional resilience by reducing stress, enhancing mood, and promoting mental clarity. Here's how walking helps foster emotional strength and resilience:

- **Reducing Cortisol Levels**: Cortisol is the body's primary stress hormone, and elevated levels can lead to feelings of anxiety, tension, and irritability. Walking helps reduce cortisol levels by promoting relaxation and lowering the body's stress response. Over time, regular walking helps your body become less reactive to stress, making it easier to manage daily pressures.

- **Stimulating Endorphin Release**: Walking stimulates the release of endorphins, the brain's natural "feel-good" chemicals. Endorphins help improve your mood, reduce pain, and create a sense of well-being. This endorphin boost enhances emotional resilience by helping you stay positive, even when facing challenges.

- **Improving Sleep Quality**: Quality sleep is essential for emotional resilience, as it allows your brain to recover from the day's stressors and regulate mood. Walking improves sleep by reducing stress, promoting relaxation, and helping regulate your body's sleep-wake cycle. Better sleep means better emotional regulation and mental clarity, which are key components of resilience.

- **Increasing Serotonin and Dopamine**: Walking increases the production of serotonin and dopamine, neurotransmitters that are associated with happiness, motivation, and emotional balance. Higher levels of these neurotransmitters help you stay emotionally grounded and maintain a positive outlook, even in difficult situations.

Walking as a Stress Management Tool

One of the most significant benefits of walking for emotional resilience is its ability to help you manage stress. Whether you're dealing with work pressures, personal challenges, or emotional turmoil, walking provides a healthy outlet for stress relief.

Here's how walking helps reduce and manage stress:

- **Physical Release of Tension**: Stress often manifests physically, leading to muscle tension, headaches, and fatigue. Walking helps release this built-up tension by encouraging your muscles to relax and promoting circulation. The rhythmic movement of walking can be meditative, allowing your mind to focus on the present moment and release worries.

- **Distraction and Mental Clarity**: Walking provides a mental break from stressors by shifting your focus away from problems and allowing your mind to clear. This distraction gives your brain a chance to reset, helping you return to challenges with a fresh perspective and renewed mental clarity. Many people find that walking helps them come up with solutions to problems they couldn't resolve while sitting still.

- **Mindfulness and Stress Reduction**: Walking is an excellent opportunity to practice mindfulness, which is the act of being fully present in the moment. Mindful walking helps reduce stress by encouraging you to focus on your breath, your surroundings, and your body's movements, rather than ruminating on stressful thoughts. This mindfulness practice promotes relaxation and emotional balance, making it easier to manage stress effectively.

- **Promoting Emotional Release**: Walking provides a safe space for emotional release, allowing you to process difficult emotions like anger, frustration, or sadness. Physical movement helps release emotional energy, preventing it from building up and causing mental exhaustion. After a walk, many people feel calmer, more balanced, and better equipped to handle their emotions.

Walking for a Positive Mindset

In addition to managing stress, walking helps foster a positive mindset by boosting mood, enhancing mental clarity, and encouraging gratitude. The simple act of moving your body outdoors can significantly improve your mental outlook and create a sense of joy and contentment.

Here's how walking helps promote a positive mindset:

- **Boosting Mood and Easing Depression**: Walking has been shown to reduce symptoms of depression by increasing the production of mood-enhancing neurotransmitters like serotonin and endorphins. Regular physical activity helps alleviate feelings of sadness or hopelessness and creates a more positive mental state. Many people find that walking outdoors, in particular, has a powerful uplifting effect on their mood.

- **Encouraging Gratitude and Mindfulness**: Walking outdoors gives you the opportunity to connect with nature and appreciate the world around you. This practice of mindful walking encourages a sense of gratitude, which is closely linked to emotional resilience. By focusing on the beauty of your surroundings, you can cultivate a more positive and grateful mindset, even when dealing with challenges.

- **Reducing Negative Thought Patterns**: Negative thought patterns, such as rumination or catastrophizing, can contribute to feelings of anxiety and emotional overwhelm. Walking helps break these patterns by redirecting your focus and encouraging you to engage in the present moment. This mental shift allows you to approach problems with a clearer, more balanced perspective, making it easier to stay positive and resilient.

- **Promoting a Sense of Accomplishment**: Setting and achieving small goals, such as completing your daily walk, provides a sense of accomplishment that boosts self-esteem and reinforces a positive mindset. Walking regularly builds confidence in your ability to take control of your physical and mental health, fostering a greater sense of empowerment and resilience.

Using Walking to Build Emotional Resilience: Practical Tips

To get the most emotional benefits from walking, it's important to incorporate it into your daily routine in a way that supports your mental and emotional well-being. Here are some practical tips for using walking to build emotional resilience and foster a positive mindset:

1. **Walk Consistently**
   Consistency is key to building emotional resilience through walking. Aim to walk 4 miles a day, most days of the week, to keep your stress levels in check and maintain a positive outlook. Even on days when you feel overwhelmed, taking a short walk can help you reset and regain emotional balance.

2. **Practice Mindful Walking**
   Incorporate mindfulness into your walks by focusing on the present moment. Pay attention to your breath, the feeling of your

feet hitting the ground, and the sights and sounds around you. Practicing mindful walking helps reduce stress, clear your mind, and promote a sense of calm and well-being.

3.   **Use Walking as a Mental Break**
     If you're feeling stressed or overwhelmed, use walking as a mental break to clear your head and reset your emotions. A 10-15 minute walk can provide the mental space you need to process difficult emotions and return to your tasks with greater clarity and focus.

4.   **Walk in Nature**
     Walking in natural environments, such as parks, forests, or near bodies of water, enhances the emotional benefits of walking. Being in nature has been shown to reduce stress, improve mood, and promote feelings of peace and relaxation. Whenever possible, choose outdoor walking routes that allow you to connect with nature.

5.   **Reflect on Gratitude During Your Walks**
     Use your walking time to reflect on the things you're grateful for. Gratitude has been shown to improve emotional resilience by fostering a positive mindset and reducing negative thought patterns. As you walk, think about the things in your life that bring you joy, comfort, and fulfillment.

6.   **Set Intentions for Your Walks**
     Before each walk, set an intention to focus on a specific area of emotional resilience, such as reducing stress, boosting mood, or finding mental clarity. Setting an intention helps guide your thoughts during the walk and ensures that your walking routine

supports your emotional well-being.

The Long-Term Benefits of Walking for Emotional Resilience

The emotional resilience you build through walking extends far beyond immediate stress relief. Over time, consistent walking helps you develop the mental strength and emotional stability needed to navigate life's challenges with confidence and grace. Walking enhances your ability to recover from setbacks, maintain a positive outlook, and manage stress effectively, leading to long-term emotional health.

As you continue walking regularly, you'll notice that you're better able to handle difficult situations, regulate your emotions, and stay mentally strong in the face of adversity. The mental and emotional strength you build through walking will serve as a foundation for a healthier, happier, and more resilient life.

Conclusion: Walking for Mental Strength and Positivity

Walking 4 miles a day is a powerful tool for building emotional resilience, reducing stress, and fostering a positive mindset. By reducing cortisol levels, stimulating endorphin release, and promoting mental clarity, walking helps you stay mentally strong and emotionally balanced, even in the face of life's challenges.

Chapter 22: Boosting Creativity – How Walking Unlocks New Ideas and Insights

Creativity is the ability to think in new ways, solve problems, and generate original ideas. Whether you're an artist, writer, entrepreneur, or simply looking for creative solutions to everyday challenges, tapping into your creativity can help you approach problems with fresh perspectives. Walking 4 miles a day is one of the most effective ways to stimulate creativity and unlock new ideas. Research shows that walking enhances cognitive flexibility, promotes divergent thinking, and helps break mental blocks, making it a powerful tool for creativity.

In this chapter, we'll explore how walking boosts creativity, why it's so effective for generating new ideas, and practical strategies for using walking to enhance your creative process.

How Walking Enhances Creativity

Walking stimulates the brain in a way that enhances creative thinking. While walking, the brain enters a relaxed, yet focused state that encourages new ideas and connections. This blend of physical movement and mental relaxation allows for more flexible thinking, which is key to creativity.

Here's how walking boosts creativity:

- **Promoting Divergent Thinking**: Creativity often involves divergent thinking, which is the ability to generate multiple ideas or solutions to a problem. Walking encourages divergent thinking by freeing the mind from distractions and allowing thoughts to flow more naturally. When walking, your brain is more likely to make novel connections, leading to creative insights.

- **Activating Both Hemispheres of the Brain**: Walking engages both the left and right hemispheres of the brain, which are responsible for different types of thinking. The left hemisphere is more analytical, while the right hemisphere is associated with creativity and intuition. Walking helps balance these two modes of thinking, allowing you to approach problems from both a logical and creative perspective.

- **Reducing Mental Blocks**: Mental blocks occur when you're stuck on a problem and can't seem to generate new ideas. Walking helps break through mental blocks by shifting your focus away from the problem and giving your brain a chance to relax. This mental reset allows you to return to the problem with fresh eyes and new ideas.

- **Improving Cognitive Flexibility**: Cognitive flexibility is the brain's ability to switch between different ideas or perspectives. Walking improves cognitive flexibility by stimulating brain activity and encouraging open-minded thinking. This flexibility makes it easier to think creatively, solve problems, and generate innovative ideas.

The Science Behind Walking and Creativity

Research has shown a strong link between walking and increased creativity. One notable study conducted by Stanford University found that walking boosts creative output by an average of 60% compared to sitting. The study revealed that participants who walked—either indoors on a treadmill or outdoors—produced more creative responses to problem-solving tasks than those who remained seated.

This increase in creativity is attributed to several factors:

- **Increased Oxygen and Blood Flow**: Walking increases blood flow to the brain, which delivers more oxygen and nutrients to brain cells. This enhanced circulation helps improve brain function and mental clarity, making it easier to generate new ideas.

- **Relaxation of the Mind**: Walking helps put the brain into a relaxed, yet alert state known as "flow," where creativity thrives. This state of mind allows ideas to flow more freely without the constraints of stress or overthinking. Many people find that their best ideas come when they're not actively trying to think of solutions but instead letting their minds wander.

- **Engagement with the Environment**: Walking outdoors provides exposure to new stimuli, such as different sights, sounds, and smells. This sensory engagement stimulates the brain and encourages creative thinking by offering fresh perspectives and inspiration from the environment.

Walking to Solve Problems and Generate New Ideas

Walking is a highly effective tool for solving problems and generating new ideas, whether you're brainstorming for a project, trying to come up with a creative solution, or working through a mental block. The act of walking helps you distance yourself from the problem, giving your brain the mental space it needs to think more creatively.

Here's how to use walking to solve problems and generate new ideas:

- **Break from Focused Thinking**: When you're stuck on a problem, it's often because you're too focused on a specific solution or approach. Walking helps you step away from the problem and engage in a more relaxed, open form of thinking. By giving your brain a break from focused thinking, you allow new ideas to surface naturally.

- **Encouraging Mind-Wandering**: Creative insights often come when you're not actively thinking about the problem. Walking encourages mind-wandering, a mental state in which your thoughts flow freely and spontaneously. This unstructured thinking helps you make unexpected connections, leading to creative breakthroughs.

- **Creating Mental Space**: Walking helps clear mental clutter, making room for new ideas to emerge. When your mind is overloaded with information or stress, it can be difficult to think creatively. Walking provides the mental space needed for reflection, allowing you to approach problems with fresh perspectives.

- **Boosting Confidence in Ideas**: Walking not only helps generate new ideas but also boosts confidence in those ideas. The physical movement and increased blood flow during walking can enhance your sense of motivation and clarity, making you more confident in your ability to act on creative insights.

Walking to Enhance Creative Projects

Whether you're an artist, writer, musician, or entrepreneur, walking can enhance your creative process by providing fresh inspiration, mental clarity, and a break from routine. Many famous creators, from writers like Virginia Woolf to inventors like Steve Jobs, have used walking as part of their creative routine to generate new ideas and overcome creative blocks.

Here's how walking can enhance your creative projects:

- **Generating Inspiration**: Walking, especially in nature or new environments, provides a source of inspiration that can fuel your creative work. The sights, sounds, and sensory experiences of walking outdoors can spark new ideas, help you see things from a different perspective, and provide creative material for your projects.

- **Overcoming Creative Blocks**: Creative blocks can be frustrating and hinder your progress on a project. Walking helps break through these blocks by stimulating creative thinking and allowing ideas to flow more freely. If you're feeling stuck, taking a walk can help reset your mind and provide new insights for moving forward.

- **Improving Focus on Creative Tasks**: Walking improves mental clarity and focus, which can help you concentrate on creative tasks more effectively. After a walk, you may find that you're better able to focus on your work and approach it with renewed energy and enthusiasm.

- **Creating a Routine for Creativity**: Incorporating walking into your daily routine can help establish a creative rhythm, where you regularly take time to reflect, brainstorm, and generate new ideas. Many creative professionals find that walking at the same time each day helps them stay mentally fresh and productive.

Practical Tips for Using Walking to Boost Creativity

To maximize the creative benefits of walking, it's helpful to approach your walks with intention and mindfulness. Here are some practical tips for using walking to enhance creativity:

1. **Walk in New Environments**
    Walking in new or unfamiliar environments helps stimulate your brain with fresh stimuli. If possible, explore different routes, parks, or neighborhoods to provide new visual and sensory experiences. These novel environments can inspire creativity and help you think outside the box.

2. **Alternate Between Focus and Mind-Wandering**
    While walking, alternate between focused thinking and allowing your mind to wander. Start by focusing on the problem or project you're working on, then let your thoughts drift and see where they take you. This balance between focused and open thinking is key to generating creative insights.

3. **Walk Without Distractions**
    Avoid distractions like listening to podcasts or music while walking if your goal is to enhance creativity. Allow your mind to be free of external input so that it can focus on generating new ideas. If you find that silence helps you think more clearly, take a quiet walk in nature or a peaceful environment.

4. **Use Walking as Part of a Brainstorming Session**
    If you're brainstorming for a project or trying to solve a problem, use walking as part of the process. Take breaks during brainstorming sessions to go for a walk, allowing your mind to reset and come up with new ideas. You can also bring a notebook or voice recorder to capture any ideas that come to you during the

walk.

5. **Incorporate Walking into Your Creative Routine**
   Make walking a regular part of your creative routine by
   scheduling daily walks as time for reflection and idea generation.
   Whether it's a morning walk to start your day or an afternoon
   break to clear your mind, regular walking can help keep your
   creativity flowing consistently.

The Long-Term Benefits of Walking for Creativity

The creative benefits of walking are not just immediate; they also build
over time. By making walking a regular part of your routine, you'll
experience sustained improvements in creativity, mental clarity, and
problem-solving abilities. Walking helps train your brain to think more
flexibly and approach challenges with an open, innovative mindset.

Over time, regular walking can help you break through creative blocks
more easily, generate new ideas more consistently, and approach your
projects with greater confidence and focus. The more you walk, the more
you'll notice that creative insights come to you naturally, whether during
or after your walks.

Conclusion: Walking to Unlock Creativity and New Ideas

Walking 4 miles a day is one of the most effective ways to boost
creativity, unlock new ideas, and break through mental blocks. By
promoting divergent thinking, reducing mental fatigue, and improving
cognitive flexibility, walking helps you approach problems with fresh
perspectives and generate creative insights.

Chapter 23: Goal Setting – Walking for Purpose and Achievement

Setting and achieving goals is an essential part of leading a purposeful, fulfilling life. Goals give us direction, motivation, and a sense of accomplishment. Whether you're working toward personal development, fitness milestones, or professional success, having clear goals helps you stay focused and on track. Walking 4 miles a day is not only an effective way to maintain physical health, but it can also be a powerful tool for setting and achieving goals in all areas of life.

In this chapter, we'll explore how walking can help you set meaningful goals, maintain motivation, and create a sense of purpose. You'll also learn strategies for using walking to achieve goals—both big and small—and how the practice of walking can help you build resilience and perseverance.

The Connection Between Walking and Goal Setting

Walking offers a unique opportunity to reflect, plan, and strategize around your personal and professional goals. The mental clarity that comes from walking can help you organize your thoughts, set clear intentions, and build a pathway toward achievement.

Here's how walking supports goal setting:

- **Creating Mental Space for Reflection**: Walking gives you time to step away from distractions and reflect on what's important to you. This reflective space allows you to think deeply about your goals, why they matter, and how you can achieve them. Many people find that walking helps them clarify their priorities and gain insight into the steps they need to take to reach their objectives.

- **Boosting Motivation and Focus**: Walking releases endorphins, which improve mood and boost motivation. When you feel good physically and mentally, you're more likely to stay motivated and focused on your goals. Walking can also provide a sense of accomplishment in itself, reinforcing your commitment to other goals.

- **Strengthening Discipline and Routine**: Committing to walking 4 miles a day helps build discipline and consistency, two key ingredients for achieving goals. The daily practice of walking teaches you to follow through on commitments and create a routine that supports long-term success. These habits can then be applied to other areas of your life, helping you stay focused on your goals.

- **Providing a Break for Problem Solving**: When you're faced with obstacles or challenges in your goal-setting journey, walking can help clear your mind and provide a fresh perspective. The act of walking allows your brain to relax, making it easier to solve problems and find creative solutions.

How Walking Helps You Achieve Fitness and Health Goals

One of the most obvious ways walking supports goal setting is through fitness and health. Walking 4 miles a day can help you achieve a wide range of health-related goals, whether you're looking to lose weight, improve cardiovascular health, or increase stamina. The consistency of walking builds momentum toward these goals, making them more attainable.

Here's how walking helps you achieve your health and fitness goals:

- **Tracking Progress**: Walking provides an easy way to track your progress toward fitness goals. By measuring distance, time, or steps, you can see tangible improvements in your endurance and fitness levels over time. This sense of progress reinforces your motivation to continue walking and stay on track with your goals.

- **Creating Measurable Milestones**: Walking allows you to set measurable goals, such as walking a certain distance, increasing your walking speed, or reaching a specific number of steps each day. These smaller milestones help break down larger fitness goals into achievable steps, making it easier to stay committed and track your success.

- **Building Physical and Mental Resilience**: The consistency of walking strengthens both your body and your mind, helping you build the resilience needed to tackle larger health challenges. Walking promotes cardiovascular health, builds muscle endurance, and supports weight management, all of which contribute to achieving your overall fitness goals.

- **Staying Motivated and Energized**: Walking boosts energy levels, reduces stress, and improves mood, all of which help you stay motivated to pursue your health and fitness goals. The physical and mental benefits of walking provide the momentum you need to keep moving forward, even when challenges arise.

Using Walking as a Tool for Personal and Professional Goal Achievement

Walking is not just a physical activity—it can also be a tool for achieving personal and professional goals. The mental clarity and focus that come from walking can help you plan, strategize, and stay motivated as you work toward your goals.

Here's how walking can support goal achievement in various areas of life:

- **Personal Growth Goals**: Walking provides a time for introspection and self-reflection, helping you think about personal growth goals such as improving self-discipline, building better habits, or learning new skills. Use your walks to reflect on where you want to grow, set intentions for personal development, and brainstorm actionable steps to move forward.

- **Career and Professional Goals**: Many successful professionals use walking as a way to think through career challenges, strategize for business goals, and stay focused on long-term objectives. Walking allows you to step away from your desk, clear your mind, and think creatively about how to achieve your career goals. It's also a great way to process feedback, reflect on your progress, and set new professional milestones.

- **Creative and Project Goals**: If you're working on a creative project or personal passion, walking can help you stay motivated and inspired. Use your walks to brainstorm ideas, outline steps, and develop a plan of action for achieving your creative goals. Walking boosts creativity and problem-solving, making it an ideal activity for overcoming creative blocks and finding new perspectives on your projects.

- **Relationship and Social Goals**: Walking can also support your goals related to relationships and social connections. Walking with a partner, friend, or group allows you to spend quality time together while working toward health and fitness goals. It also provides an opportunity to reflect on how you can improve your relationships, strengthen your communication skills, or set goals for personal connection.

Goal Setting and Visualization During Walks

One of the most powerful aspects of walking for goal achievement is the opportunity it provides for visualization. Visualization is the process of mentally picturing yourself achieving your goals, which can help increase motivation and clarify your path to success.

Here's how to use walking to set goals and visualize success:

- **Set Clear Goals**: As you walk, think about the specific goals you want to achieve, whether they're related to health, career, personal growth, or relationships. Be as clear and detailed as possible when defining your goals. For example, instead of simply saying, "I want to be healthier," set a goal like, "I want to lose 10 pounds in three months by walking daily and improving my diet."

- **Visualize the Process**: While walking, visualize the steps you need to take to achieve your goals. Picture yourself completing each step and overcoming obstacles along the way. This mental rehearsal helps reinforce your commitment to your goals and gives you a clear sense of the actions required to achieve them.

- **Imagine the End Result**: Visualize yourself achieving your goal and experiencing the rewards of your success. Imagine how it will feel to accomplish your goal, whether it's crossing the finish line at a race, reaching a career milestone, or building stronger relationships. This positive visualization reinforces your motivation and helps you stay focused on the bigger picture.

- **Reflect on Your Progress**: Use your walks as an opportunity to reflect on the progress you've made toward your goals. Celebrate small wins and think about how far you've come, even if you're not at the finish line yet. Reflecting on progress keeps you motivated and encourages perseverance.

Staying Motivated and Accountable Through Walking

One of the challenges of goal setting is staying motivated and accountable over time. Walking can help you stay on track by providing a daily routine that reinforces your commitment to your goals.

Here's how to use walking to maintain motivation and accountability:

- **Set Daily Walking Goals**: Make walking 4 miles a day a non-negotiable part of your routine. Setting a daily walking goal creates consistency and builds momentum, helping you stay motivated to pursue your larger goals. Tracking your daily walking progress—whether through a fitness tracker or journal—can also provide a sense of accountability and accomplishment.

- **Celebrate Milestones**: As you work toward your goals, celebrate small milestones along the way. Each time you reach a new walking distance, improve your speed, or make progress toward a non-fitness goal, take a moment to acknowledge your success. Celebrating milestones helps reinforce your motivation and reminds you that you're on the right path.

- **Use Walking to Stay Focused**: When you feel like you're losing motivation or getting off track with your goals, use walking as a tool to refocus. Walking gives you the mental space to reset, reevaluate your priorities, and recommit to your goals. It also helps relieve stress and anxiety, which can often interfere with motivation.

- **Involve Others for Accountability**: Walking with friends, family members, or a group can help you stay accountable to your goals. Sharing your goals with others and walking together provides a built-in support system, making it easier to stay on track. Plus, having a walking buddy adds an element of fun and social connection to your goal-setting journey.

The Long-Term Benefits of Using Walking for Goal Achievement

Walking regularly not only helps you achieve your short-term goals but also provides long-term benefits for personal development and success. The discipline, focus, and resilience you build through walking can be applied to all areas of your life, helping you stay committed to your goals and continue growing as a person.

By making walking a part of your goal-setting process, you'll experience a sense of accomplishment, increased mental clarity, and the motivation to keep pushing toward your dreams. Over time, the consistency and focus you develop through walking will help you achieve even your most ambitious goals.

Conclusion: Walking for Purpose and Achievement

Walking 4 miles a day is a powerful tool for setting and achieving goals in all areas of life. By providing mental clarity, boosting motivation, and reinforcing discipline, walking helps you stay focused on your objectives and build the resilience needed to reach your goals. Whether you're working toward fitness milestones, personal growth, or professional success, walking gives you the mental and physical stamina to keep moving forward.

Chapter 24: Building Self-Discipline – Walking for Routine and Commitment

Self-discipline is the cornerstone of success in any area of life. It's the ability to stay committed to your goals, follow through on your promises, and maintain focus even when motivation wanes. Building self-discipline takes practice, but once developed, it provides the foundation for long-term achievement and personal growth. Walking 4 miles a day is an excellent way to cultivate self-discipline. The consistency required to maintain a daily walking routine helps strengthen your ability to stick to your commitments, both in fitness and in other areas of your life.

In this chapter, we'll explore how walking helps build self-discipline, why routine is so important for long-term success, and practical tips for using walking as a tool to develop stronger discipline in all areas of life.

The Role of Self-Discipline in Success

Self-discipline is the ability to control impulses, stay focused on your goals, and take consistent action, even when it's difficult. It's what helps you resist distractions, overcome obstacles, and maintain the habits necessary to achieve long-term success. While motivation can be fleeting, self-discipline is the force that keeps you moving forward, especially on days when you don't feel like it.

Here's why self-discipline is essential for success:

- **Consistency is Key**: Whether you're working toward fitness goals, career milestones, or personal growth, consistency is what ultimately leads to success. Self-discipline ensures that you take action every day, even when progress feels slow. By staying consistent, you build momentum and create lasting change.

- **Overcoming Short-Term Impulses**: Self-discipline helps you resist the temptation of short-term gratification in favor of long-term rewards. This might mean choosing a walk over watching TV, or working on a project instead of scrolling through social media. Self-discipline gives you the mental strength to prioritize what truly matters over immediate comfort.

- **Building Better Habits**: Habits are the building blocks of success, and self-discipline is what helps you establish and maintain positive habits. Whether it's committing to a daily walk, sticking to a healthy diet, or managing your time effectively, self-discipline ensures that you follow through on your intentions and make those habits a part of your daily life.

How Walking Builds Self-Discipline

Walking regularly, especially when it's part of a daily routine, is a powerful way to strengthen self-discipline. The practice of committing to a 4-mile walk each day requires consistency, focus, and the ability to push through moments of discomfort—all key components of self-discipline.

Here's how walking helps build self-discipline:

- **Creating a Routine**: Walking at the same time each day helps establish a routine that becomes second nature. Once a routine is in place, it's easier to stick to your goals because you've created a structure that supports discipline. Over time, the act of walking becomes automatic, and you're less likely to skip it because it's part of your daily schedule.

- **Developing Mental Toughness**: Some days, walking 4 miles may feel easy, but other days it may be a challenge—whether due to fatigue, weather, or a busy schedule. Pushing through these moments of discomfort strengthens your mental toughness and reinforces your self-discipline. Each time you complete a walk when you didn't feel like it, you build resilience and the ability to follow through on commitments.

- **Strengthening Focus and Commitment**: Walking requires you to stay focused on your goal of completing the distance, no matter what distractions or obstacles arise. This focus and commitment to finishing your walk translate into other areas of life, helping you stay disciplined in your work, personal projects, and relationships.

- **Building Accountability**: By setting a daily walking goal and tracking your progress, you create a sense of accountability to yourself. This accountability helps reinforce discipline, as you don't want to break your streak or fall short of your goals. The more accountable you are to your walking routine, the more disciplined you become in other areas of life.

The Importance of Routine in Building Self-Discipline

Routine is a critical part of building self-discipline because it removes the need to rely on willpower alone. When you have a structured routine in place, you're less likely to make excuses or get distracted by other activities. Instead, the routine becomes a natural part of your day, making it easier to stick to your goals.

Here's why routine is so important for self-discipline:

- **Reducing Decision Fatigue**: Decision fatigue occurs when you're faced with too many choices throughout the day, leading to mental exhaustion and poor decision-making. A routine eliminates the need to make decisions about when or whether to walk, as it's already scheduled into your day. This consistency reduces decision fatigue and makes it easier to stay disciplined.

- **Building Momentum**: Once you've established a routine, each day that you stick to it builds momentum. This momentum reinforces your self-discipline and makes it easier to continue following through on your commitments. As you see progress, whether it's in your fitness or personal goals, your motivation grows, further strengthening your discipline.

- **Creating Positive Habits**: Routine helps turn actions into habits, and habits are the foundation of self-discipline. By consistently walking at the same time each day, you create a habit that becomes automatic. Once a habit is in place, it requires less effort to maintain, as your brain and body become accustomed to the routine.

- **Providing Structure and Stability**: A routine provides structure and stability, which are essential for maintaining focus and discipline. When you know exactly what needs to be done and when it needs to happen, it's easier to stay on track and avoid distractions. Walking as part of a daily routine helps anchor your day, providing a sense of purpose and direction.

Practical Tips for Using Walking to Build Self-Discipline

To use walking as a tool for building self-discipline, it's important to approach your walks with intention and consistency. Here are some practical tips for using walking to strengthen your discipline and commitment:

1. **Set a Daily Walking Goal**
   Commit to walking 4 miles a day, even if it means breaking it up
   into smaller segments throughout the day. Setting a daily goal
   helps you stay focused and gives you something to work toward
   every day. The key is consistency—aim to walk every day, even
   when you don't feel like it.

2. **Walk at the Same Time Each Day**
   Walking at the same time each day helps establish a routine that
   becomes second nature. Whether it's a morning walk to start your
   day or an evening walk to unwind, sticking to a consistent
   schedule makes it easier to build self-discipline. Over time, your
   body and mind will come to expect the walk as part of your daily
   routine.

3. **Track Your Progress**
   Tracking your daily walks—whether through a fitness app,
   journal, or calendar—provides accountability and reinforces your
   commitment to your goals. Seeing your progress in real-time
   motivates you to stay disciplined and avoid skipping your walks.
   Each day you complete a walk adds to your streak, building
   momentum and confidence.

4. **Push Through Discomfort**
   There will be days when walking feels harder than usual, whether
   due to fatigue, weather conditions, or a busy schedule. Use these
   moments as opportunities to strengthen your discipline by pushing
   through the discomfort. Each time you complete a walk under
   difficult conditions, you reinforce your ability to stay committed
   to your goals.

5. Celebrate Small Wins

Self-discipline isn't about perfection; it's about progress. Celebrate small wins along the way, whether it's completing your daily walk, increasing your walking speed, or staying consistent for a week or month. Recognizing your progress helps boost motivation and reinforces your commitment to maintaining self-discipline.

How Walking Translates to Self-Discipline in Other Areas

The self-discipline you develop through walking extends to other areas of your life, making it easier to stay committed to your goals, maintain positive habits, and manage distractions. Walking teaches you the importance of consistency, focus, and perseverance, all of which are essential for success in personal and professional pursuits.

Here's how walking can improve self-discipline in other areas of your life:

- **Work and Productivity**: The focus and discipline required to complete a daily walk can be applied to your work. Whether you're tackling a big project or managing daily tasks, the discipline you build through walking helps you stay productive, meet deadlines, and follow through on commitments.

- **Personal Development**: Walking fosters a mindset of continuous improvement and goal-setting, which can be applied to personal development. As you build discipline through walking, you'll find it easier to stay committed to other self-improvement goals, such as learning new skills, reading more, or building better habits.

- **Healthy Habits**: Walking teaches you the importance of consistency in maintaining healthy habits. The routine of walking can be a foundation for other positive habits, such as eating well, staying hydrated, and getting enough sleep. The more disciplined you become in one area, the easier it is to apply that discipline to other aspects of your health and well-being.

- **Time Management**: Committing to a daily walking routine helps improve time management by teaching you how to prioritize your time effectively. The discipline of setting aside time for walking each day translates into better time management skills, helping you stay organized and focused on your daily tasks.

The Long-Term Benefits of Building Self-Discipline Through Walking

Building self-discipline through walking has long-term benefits that extend far beyond physical fitness. The consistency, mental toughness, and accountability you develop through walking become the foundation for success in all areas of life. Over time, the discipline you build through daily walks will help you stay committed to your goals, improve your habits, and overcome obstacles with greater resilience.

As you continue walking regularly, you'll notice that self-discipline becomes easier and more natural. What once felt challenging will become part of your routine, making it easier to stay on track and achieve your goals, both in walking and in life.

Conclusion: Walking for Routine and Commitment

Walking 4 miles a day is a powerful way to build self-discipline, create a consistent routine, and stay committed to your goals. The act of walking every day strengthens your mental toughness, reinforces positive habits, and helps you stay focused on what matters most. Whether you're working on fitness goals, personal development, or professional success, the discipline you build through walking will serve as the foundation for long-term achievement.

Chapter 25: Creating Balance – Walking for a Healthy, Fulfilled Life

In our fast-paced, constantly connected world, finding balance can be challenging. Juggling work, relationships, personal growth, and self-care often feels like a struggle, leaving us feeling overwhelmed and stressed. However, creating balance in life is essential for maintaining overall well-being, happiness, and long-term success. Walking 4 miles a day can be a powerful tool for cultivating balance in your life, providing time for reflection, relaxation, and mental clarity, while also enhancing your physical health.

In this final chapter, we'll explore how walking helps create a balanced life, how to integrate walking into your daily routine to promote physical and emotional well-being, and practical strategies for using walking to achieve a healthier, more fulfilled life.

Why Balance is Essential for Well-Being

Balance means finding a harmony between different aspects of your life —work, relationships, health, personal development, and leisure—so that no one area overwhelms the others. A balanced life leads to greater happiness, better health, and reduced stress, allowing you to feel more grounded and fulfilled.

Here's why balance is crucial for overall well-being:

- **Reducing Stress and Burnout**: When life is out of balance, we often experience stress and burnout. Too much focus on work or personal responsibilities can leave little room for relaxation or self-care, leading to physical and emotional exhaustion. Balance helps reduce stress by ensuring that you make time for rest, reflection, and rejuvenation.

- **Improving Relationships**: Creating balance in life allows you to prioritize relationships with family, friends, and loved ones. When you make time for meaningful connections, you improve the quality of your relationships and experience deeper emotional fulfillment.

- **Promoting Mental Clarity**: A balanced life helps prevent mental overload, making it easier to think clearly and make better decisions. Balance ensures that you're not overwhelmed by one area of life, such as work, and that you have the mental space to reflect, set goals, and pursue personal growth.

- **Maintaining Physical Health**: Balance includes taking care of your body through regular exercise, a healthy diet, and adequate rest. When life is out of balance, it's easy to neglect physical health. Incorporating activities like walking into your routine helps maintain physical well-being and creates a healthy foundation for the rest of your life.

How Walking Promotes a Balanced Life

Walking is one of the most accessible and effective ways to bring balance to your life. By dedicating time each day to walking, you create a space for physical activity, mental relaxation, and emotional reflection. This daily practice can help you manage stress, improve focus, and ensure that you're taking care of both your body and mind.

Here's how walking promotes balance:

- **Providing Time for Self-Care**: Walking gives you dedicated time for self-care, a crucial aspect of maintaining balance. During your walks, you're focusing on your physical health while also

allowing your mind to relax. This self-care practice helps recharge
your energy and ensures that you're not neglecting your own well-
being in the midst of daily responsibilities.

- **Encouraging Mental and Emotional Reflection**: Walking
  creates mental space for reflection, helping you process your
  thoughts and emotions. This time allows you to think about what's
  working in your life, what might need adjustment, and how you
  can better manage your priorities. Walking helps create clarity,
  making it easier to strike a balance between competing demands.

- **Integrating Physical Activity**: Physical health is a key
  component of a balanced life, and walking ensures that you're
  getting regular exercise without the need for a gym or complex
  workout routine. The simplicity of walking allows you to fit
  physical activity into your day, regardless of your schedule,
  helping you maintain balance between work, personal
  commitments, and self-care.

- **Creating a Break from Technology**: In a world dominated by
  screens and constant connectivity, walking provides a much-
  needed break from technology. Stepping away from your phone,
  computer, or TV during your walk helps you reconnect with
  nature, clear your mind, and reduce mental fatigue. This break
  helps restore balance by encouraging mindfulness and presence in
  the moment.

- **Enhancing Sleep and Relaxation**: Regular walking promotes
  better sleep, which is essential for maintaining balance in life.
  Quality sleep helps you manage stress, improve focus, and
  maintain emotional stability. Walking also encourages relaxation
  by reducing cortisol levels and promoting the release of

endorphins, helping you unwind at the end of the day.

Finding Balance Through Walking: Practical Tips

To use walking as a tool for creating balance in your life, it's important to approach your walks with mindfulness and intention. Here are some practical tips for using walking to cultivate a healthier, more balanced lifestyle:

1. **Schedule Walking as "Me Time"**
   Treat your daily walks as sacred time for yourself. Block off time in your schedule, whether it's in the morning, during lunch, or in the evening, to ensure that walking becomes a priority. This dedicated "me time" helps create balance by giving you space to focus on your well-being without distractions.

2. **Use Walking to Reflect on Priorities**
   During your walks, take time to reflect on your priorities and how you're allocating your time and energy. Are there areas of your life that feel out of balance? What can you adjust to create more harmony? Use this time for self-reflection, and consider journaling after your walk to capture any insights or ideas that come to mind.

3. **Walk in Nature Whenever Possible**
   Walking in nature has been shown to enhance mental and emotional well-being, making it an ideal way to create balance. If possible, walk in parks, forests, or along scenic routes to reconnect with the natural world. Nature walks provide a calming, grounding experience that helps reduce stress and restore balance to your mind and body.

4.   **Walk with a Friend or Loved One**
Walking with others can help strengthen relationships and create balance between social connections and personal well-being. Invite a friend, family member, or partner to join you on your walks, allowing you to bond while also taking care of your physical health. Social walks provide an opportunity to connect meaningfully with others, improving your emotional well-being.

5.   **Listen to Your Body**
Walking is a gentle form of exercise, but it's still important to listen to your body and adjust your pace or distance as needed. If you're feeling fatigued or stressed, a slower, shorter walk may be more beneficial than pushing yourself to walk faster or farther. Creating balance means respecting your body's needs and ensuring that your walks are restorative rather than depleting.

Achieving Long-Term Balance Through Walking

Walking regularly not only promotes immediate feelings of balance and well-being, but it also supports long-term harmony in your life. By making walking a consistent part of your routine, you build a foundation for physical, mental, and emotional health that sustains you over time. Walking helps prevent burnout, reduces stress, and ensures that you have the energy and clarity to manage life's demands with ease.

Here's how walking helps achieve long-term balance:

- **Sustaining Physical Health**: Regular walking keeps your body strong, mobile, and energized, providing the physical foundation needed to handle life's challenges. By staying active through walking, you reduce the risk of chronic illnesses, improve cardiovascular health, and maintain flexibility and strength as you age.

- **Maintaining Mental Clarity**: Walking helps prevent mental overload by giving you regular time to clear your mind, reflect on your priorities, and gain perspective. Over time, this practice of mental clarity allows you to manage stress more effectively, make better decisions, and stay focused on what truly matters.

- **Fostering Emotional Resilience**: Walking enhances emotional well-being by reducing anxiety, improving mood, and promoting relaxation. This emotional resilience helps you stay calm and centered, even when life feels chaotic or stressful. The more you walk, the more emotionally balanced and grounded you'll feel.

- **Creating a Lifestyle of Mindfulness and Presence**: By incorporating walking into your daily routine, you cultivate a lifestyle that values mindfulness, presence, and self-care. Walking encourages you to slow down, tune in to your surroundings, and appreciate the moment. This practice of mindfulness helps you stay balanced, even in the midst of a busy schedule.

Conclusion: Walking for a Healthy, Fulfilled Life

Walking 4 miles a day is one of the most effective ways to create balance, maintain health, and live a fulfilled life. By providing time for self-care, reflection, and relaxation, walking helps you manage stress, improve physical and mental well-being, and ensure that you're living in harmony with your goals and priorities.

Before starting any physical exercise program consult your Doctor and make sure it's right for you.

Good Luck!

Please return to "4 Miles A Day" Amazon page and leave a review and thank you.